Cambridge Elements ≡

Elements in England in the Early Medieval World
edited by
Megan Cavell
University of Birmingham
Rory Naismith
University of Cambridge
Winfried Rudolf
University of Göttingen
Emily V. Thornbury
Yale University

HEALTH AND THE BODY IN EARLY MEDIEVAL ENGLAND

Caroline Batten
University of Pennsylvania

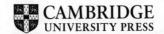

CAMBRIDGE
UNIVERSITY PRESS

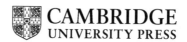

Shaftesbury Road, Cambridge CB2 8EA, United Kingdom

One Liberty Plaza, 20th Floor, New York, NY 10006, USA

477 Williamstown Road, Port Melbourne, VIC 3207, Australia

314–321, 3rd Floor, Plot 3, Splendor Forum, Jasola District Centre, New Delhi – 110025, India

103 Penang Road, #05–06/07, Visioncrest Commercial, Singapore 238467

Cambridge University Press is part of Cambridge University Press & Assessment, a department of the University of Cambridge.

We share the University's mission to contribute to society through the pursuit of education, learning and research at the highest international levels of excellence.

www.cambridge.org
Information on this title: www.cambridge.org/9781009500203

DOI: 10.1017/9781009246248

First published 2024

A catalogue record for this publication is available from the British Library.

ISBN 978-1-009-50020-3 Hardback
ISBN 978-1-009-24625-5 Paperback
ISSN 2632-203X (online)
ISSN 2632-2021 (print)

Cambridge University Press & Assessment has no responsibility for the persistence or accuracy of URLs for external or third-party internet websites referred to in this publication and does not guarantee that any content on such websites is, or will remain, accurate or appropriate.

Health and the Body in Early Medieval England

Elements in England in the Early Medieval World

DOI: 10.1017/9781009246248
First published online: December 2024

Caroline Batten
University of Pennsylvania

Author for correspondence: Caroline Batten, battenc@english.upenn.edu

Abstract: This Element explores ideas about the sick and healthy body in early medieval England from the seventh to the eleventh centuries, proposing that surviving Old English texts offer consistent and coherent ideas about how human bodies work and how disease operates. A close examination of these texts illuminates the ways early medieval people thought about their embodied selves and the place of humanity in a fallen world populated by hostile supernatural forces. This Element offers a comprehensive and accessible introduction to medical practice and writing in England before the Norman Conquest, draws on dozens of remedies, charms, and prayers to illustrate cultural concepts of sickness and health, provides a detailed discussion of the way impairment and disability were treated in literature and experienced by individuals, and concludes with a case study of a saint who died of a devastating illness while fighting demons in the fens of East Anglia.

Keywords: Old English, history of medicine, history of the body, disability, St Guthlac

ISBNs: 9781009500203 (HB), 9781009246255 (PB), 9781009246248 (OC)
ISSNs: 2632-203X (online), 2632-2021 (print)

Contents

Introduction

An eleventh-century remedy for sickness caused by the influence of elves and the temptations of devils instructs the practitioner to write a number of biblical verses across a dish used for bearing the Eucharist, create a tonic of herbs and wine, wash the writing ink off the dish into the drink, have multiple masses and psalms said over the concoction, and then administer the drink to a sick patient, purifying them from the inside out.[1] This Element offers an introduction to ideas about sick and healthy bodies that gave rise to this complex remedy and others like it in early medieval England – that is, the period between the advent of written literature in Old English in the seventh century and the Norman Conquest in the eleventh. This Element necessarily focuses most closely on the latter half of that period, when the extant Old English medical texts were written and copied.

At this time, medical practice in Europe was largely dependent upon both vernacular traditions of which only traces survive, and the dissemination of late antique Latin medical texts within and between monastic intellectual centres – modes of medical practice that mutually influenced one another. The vast majority of celebrated medicine written in Greek and Arabic would only become available in Western Europe in the twelfth century, after scholars from the Arabic-speaking world translated these texts into Latin. The first medical school in Europe, the famed Schola Medica Salernitana, would not rise to prominence – and establish a set medical curriculum used across the European continent – until that time.

Old English medical literature is one of the few, and by far the largest, surviving corpuses of vernacular medicine from the early medieval period in Europe. Both Old English remedies without identifiable Latin sources – likely representatives of a medical tradition specific to early medieval England – and the numerous English translations of Latin remedies that adapt and alter their source material, offer an unusual degree of insight into how patients and practitioners in the pre-Conquest period thought about disease, what constituted medicine, and how that medicine worked. The themes and anxieties that animate the Old English medical corpus as well as Old English literary depictions of the sick body persisted into late medieval and early modern English medicine, transmuting with time to accommodate new cultural and political concerns. These themes are reflected in the smaller, more enigmatic medical corpuses of related languages like Old Norse and Old High German.[2] And as a result, these Old English texts

---

[1] London, British Library, Harley MS 585 ff. 137r–138r. *Lacnunga* no. 29. All citations from the *Lacnunga* are taken from Pettit, *Anglo-Saxon Remedies*. For those wishing to consult the original, the manuscript folio numbers for every *Lacnunga* remedy cited here are given in the footnotes of Pettit's edition.

[2] For introductions to Old Norse medical material, see Jesch and Lee, 'Healing Runes'; Mitchell, 'Leechbooks'. For medieval German, see Murdoch, 'Charms'.

offer scholars some of the clearest possible access to the ways early medieval English people understood the structure, functions, strengths, and vulnerabilities of their bodies.

This Element begins with an overview of what is currently known about medical practice in England in the early medieval period, before turning to a detailed discussion of the ways Old English medical texts conceive of and depict sickness and health. These ideas are expanded upon in an examination of attitudes towards impairment and disability in the Old English textual corpus. The Element concludes with a literary case study: an analysis of the vernacular and Latin texts describing the life and death of Guthlac of Crowland, one of England's first native saints. Reading medical and poetic texts together in this way illuminates depictions of and ideas about sickness and health that are not available to us if either genre is siloed. Across these four linked analyses, a coherent early medieval English view of the body comes into focus: one in which disease breaks open and penetrates a container-like body; one in which health is synonymous with visual wholeness; and one in which illness and impairment are understood as a loss of power in a zero-sum game, a threat to the integrity of the individual's embodied self.

Medicine in Early Medieval England

The *Old English Handbook*, a penitential containing a list of sins and the penances that should be prescribed for them, describes confession in the following way:

> Se læca þe sceal sare wunda wel gehælan, he mot habban gode sealfe
> to. Ne syndon nane swa yfele wunda swa sindon synwunda, forðam
> þurh þa forwyrð se man ecan deaðe, buton he þurh andetnesse ⁊ þurh
> geswicenesse ⁊ þurh dædbote gehæled wurðe. Þonne mot se læca
> beon wis ⁊ wær, þe ða wunda hælan sceal. Ðurh gode lare man sceal
> ærest hi lacnian ⁊ mid þam gedon þæt man aspiwe þæt attor ut þæt
> him on innan bið, þæt is þæt he geclænsige hine silfne ærost þurh
> andetnesse. Eal man sceal aspiwan synna þurh gode lare mid andetnesse,
> ealswa man unlibban deð ðurh godne drenc. . . . On wisum scrifte bið eac
> swiðe forðgelang, wislic dædbot, ealswa on godum læce bið.[3]

> If the doctor will heal painful wounds well, he must have a good salve
> for that. Nor are there any wounds as evil as the wounds of sin, because
> through these a person is annihilated in everlasting death, unless
> through confession and through abstaining and through penance he is
> healed. Then must the doctor be wise and prepared, if he will heal the

---

[3] Cambridge, Corpus Christi College MS 201, f. 121. See also Oxford, Bodleian Library, MS Laud Misc. 482, f. 2r. Text from Frantzen, 'Anglo-Saxon Penitentials'. All translations are my own unless otherwise indicated.

wounds. He should heal them first with good teaching, and so make the person vomit up that poison that is inside him, that is, that he cleanses himself first through confession. All men must vomit up sins through good teaching with confession, just as a person does poison by a good drink. ... Wise penance is greatly dependent on a wise confessor, just as [a remedy] is on a good doctor.

This metaphor, aside from telling us how seriously the early medieval English took their spiritual health, offers us some insight into what medicine was like in the pre-Conquest period. This passage suggests that a good doctor (OE *læce*) is skilled, has good judgement in selecting remedies, and has access to some sort of teaching on how to examine and treat sick patients. His professional practice includes healing wounds, but also using emetics to remove harmful substances from within the patient. A skilled doctor makes the difference between a good cure and a bad one, and such a doctor is to be respected.

The written record makes it clear that there were medical practitioners in pre-Conquest England, and that they were treated as respected authorities on the sick body. 'Lef mon læces behofað' (An injured man needs a doctor), the gnomic poem *Maxims I* tells us.[4] A speaking shield or chopping block in an Old English riddle reveals itself to be non-human by declaring that it cannot find a physician (*læcecynn*) capable of healing its wounds.[5] Homilies, sermons, and religious poetry hail God or Christ as the true doctor, capable of curing the soul.[6] Saints' lives describe the miraculous healing of intractable illnesses that even the best practitioners (OE *læceas*, Latin *medici*) are unable to treat.[7] Penitentials and lawcodes mention doctors and doctors' fees (*læce-feoh*) when discussing the legal compensation owed for inflicting a wound on another person, suggesting medics were normally available and treated injuries.[8] All of these texts, however, raise more questions than they answer. Who were doctors in pre-Conquest England? How did they gain their expertise? Where did they practice, and on whom? What kinds of wounds did they heal – and what sort of 'poison'

---

[4] *Maxims I*, l. 45. All citations of Old English poetry, unless otherwise noted, are taken from Krapp and Dobbie, ASPR.

[5] Riddle 3 (ed. Williamson), l. 10. For a full analysis, see Garner, *Hybrid Healing*, 248–71.

[6] For example, Ælfric of Eynsham, 'The Passion of St Bartholomew' (ed. Clemoes, *Homilies*, 439–50); Blickling Homily X (ed. Morris, 106–15); Vercelli Homily XI (ed. Scragg, 219–26); *Judgment Day II*, ll. 42–7, 247–50; *Lord's Prayer II*, l. 58; *Christ*, l. 1571; *Christ and Satan*, l. 588; *Solomon and Saturn I*, l. 77. For further discussion, see Kesling, *Medical Texts*, 157–67.

[7] For example, Ælfric's lives of Basil, Agatha, and Swithun (ed. Skeat, *Lives of Saints*, 50–90, 194–208, 440–70).

[8] Oxford, Bodleian Library, Junius MS 121, f. 95r (Frantzen, 'Anglo-Saxon Penitentials'); Laws of Æthelberht 62; Laws of Alfred prologue 16. All citations of Old English lawcodes are taken from Liebermann, *Die Gesetze*. For discussion, see Bolotina, 'Medicine and Society', 34; Meaney, 'Practice', 223; Banham and Voth, 'Diagnosis', 161–2. Battlefield medicine is mentioned in Bede's *Historia Ecclesiastica* (ed. Colgrave and Mynors), IV.22.

(OE *attor*, *unlibban*) was thought to be inside a sick person's body by the writer of the *Old English Handbook*? What was in this doctor's salves and drinks, how were they made, and were they effective? Evidence concerning the earliest English doctors is relatively limited and scattered across the textual and archaeological records – but piecing this evidence together creates a working picture of medical practice in England between the seventh and eleventh centuries.

Practitioners of Medicine

Much of the surviving textual evidence from the early medieval English period suggests that physicians belonged to a relatively small community of elite, educated practitioners. They could have included secular clergy and monks as well as laypeople, and it is often impossible to determine a physician's specific affiliations or personal background beyond the simple fact of their participation in powerful institutions. According to the royal biographer Asser, *medici* were present at the court of King Alfred, attempting to treat the monarch's various maladies.[9] The historian, monk, and prolific eighth-century writer Bede records several instances of high-ranking persons – abbesses, abbots, bishops – being attended by physicians in monasteries, though he never clarifies whether these physicians are monks themselves.[10] Texts from the eighth and ninth centuries, particularly Bede's *Ecclesiastical History of the English People*, mostly describe travelling clergy giving miraculous cures to sick people upon arriving in their isolated villages; for example, St Cuthbert and John of Beverley, both of whom were bishops, administer cures to sick persons while fulfilling their duties of visitation.[11] Other physicians are occasionally present in these narratives, though we hear very little about them. Bede describes monks, nuns, and guests at monasteries falling ill and receiving miraculous cures, suggesting that monasteries had some kind of sick room – and, presumably, a designated person or persons to manage the sick room and provide at least basic nursing. Some ecclesiastical centres also had direct access to written medical knowledge and an interest in applying that knowledge practically: soon after 754, Cyneheard, Bishop of Winchester, wrote a letter to Lull, Bishop of Mainz, noting that while Winchester had a number of medical books, the remedies contained therein required too many foreign ingredients, and therefore Winchester was in need of

---

[9] Asser, *Life of King Alfred* (ed. Stevenson), ch. 25.

[10] Bede, *Historia Ecclesiastica*, IV.17, IV.32; *Vita Cuthberti* (ed. Colgrave, *Two Lives*), XXIII. Illustrations of untonsured physicians appear in London, British Library, MS Sloane 2839 and Harley MS 1585, but these are twelfth-century manuscripts and the illustrations may have been copied from classical sources (MacKinney, *Illustrations*, 52–3).

[11] For a comprehensive list of all healing episodes in Bede's *Historia Ecclesiastica*, his *Vita Cuthberti*, and the anonymous *Vita Cuthberti*, see Bolotina, 'Medicine and Society', 151–6.

new medical compendia with ingredients more readily available in England.[12] There is a strong possibility that medicine was one of the subjects taught at the first school in England, established at Canterbury in the late seventh century by Archbishop Theodore (a Greek-speaking monk from Tarsus) and his colleague Hadrian (a Latin-speaking abbot from northern Africa).[13] The general picture that emerges is one of literate clergy and ecclesiastics interested in the application of medicine as an aspect of pastoral care; some medical care associated with monasteries, largely for patients affiliated with the institution; and the suggestion of some secular physicians present in the upper echelons of their communities.

We find similar evidence in texts from the tenth and eleventh centuries. One of the defining cultural developments of the tenth century was the Benedictine Reform, a religious and intellectual movement that sought to separate monks from secular clergy, bring monasteries under the Benedictine Rule and found new Benedictine institutions, and revive monastic learning and production of vernacular (i.e. English) literature. The ideal Benedictine Reform monastery possessed an infirmary, and the *Benedictine Rule* and *Regularis Concordia* charge monks with the care of their sick brethren.[14] Some English monastics evidently took an interest in medical study and application. The personal prayerbook of Ælfwine, abbot of the Winchester New Minster (d.1057), includes bloodletting information, medical prognostics, and a remedy for boils.[15] The Durham Collectar, a liturgical manuscript made for the monastic community in Chester-le-Street, features a number of tenth-century additions, including multiple prayers for healing and remedies that also appear in an Old English medical compendium usually referred to as *Lacnunga* (Remedies).[16] The Winchester monk Ælfric Bata casually mentions in his late tenth-century *Colloquy*, a Latin exercise for students designed to teach vocabulary, that the monastic herb garden is tended by a monk *medicus*, who is thought to be a good physician.[17] Abbot Baldwin of Bury St Edmunds (d.1097) was a physician to Edward the Confessor, William the Conqueror, and William Rufus, and may have established a school of medicine at the abbey.[18] While we cannot determine to what extent monastic medical practitioners – especially someone like Ælfwine, an educated non-specialist – attended patients outside the monastery or royal court, the Benedictine Reform period also saw a surge in secular clergy living amongst the laity, and laypeople increasingly relying on local minster churches for religious services and pastoral care.[19] Visitation of the sick was an

[12] Tangl, *Die Briefe*, 247.   [13] Lapidge, 'School', 50; Bede, *Historia Ecclesiastica*, V.3.

[14] *Benedicti Regula* (ed. Hanslik), ch. 36; *Regularis Concordia* (ed. Symons), chs. 10, 12.

[15] Günzel, *Prayerbook*, 1–2, 157.   [16] For texts and discussion, see Jolly, 'Prayers'.

[17] Gwara and Porter, *Conversations*, 156–7.   [18] Banham, 'Medicine at Bury'.

[19] Blair, *Church*, 368–425.

essential pastoral duty, and indeed missals and liturgical books from this period include multiple rites for such visitations and sometimes include prognostics, lunaria, and other medical information.[20] Old English medical texts copied down in the later part of the pre-Conquest period include remedies calling for the recitation of masses and liturgical prayers and the use of ecclesiastical *materia medica*, including eucharistic wafers, patens, and even church bells.[21] This combined evidence suggests that minster priests were likely candidates to be medical practitioners, although the occasional requirement to involve a 'mass-priest' (*massepreost*) in a given medical remedy suggests that the main user of the text was not assumed to be a cleric.

Most of our evidence for medical practice in early medieval England comes from the survival of the major Old English medical texts, four distinct collections of written medical material contained in manuscript copies dating to the tenth and eleventh centuries. These texts are so important they are discussed individually and in detail in a later sub-section: the Old English Herbarium Complex, an interpretative translation of multiple Latin treatises; *Bald's Leechbook*, a learned medical miscellany divided into two parts (here *I* and *II*); *Leechbook III*, a shorter miscellany appended to *Bald's Leechbook*; and the remedy collection *Lacnunga*, mentioned earlier. These compendia demonstrate that clerical and ecclesiastical interest in written medicine was, at least in certain centres of learning, profound and sustained. Much of the available evidence suggests that the practitioners who used these written Old English medical collections were hyper-educated Christians engaged in practices not only sanctioned by the church, but integrated into both monastic and clerical religious and pastoral practice. The medical and liturgical manuscripts themselves were expensive to create, must have been compiled by scholars with significant education and familiarity with Latin, and were necessarily only available to the literate. These texts may well have had a reciprocal relationship with popular medicine, but in their surviving form they are intellectual artefacts specific to a particular social class.[22] The remedies they

---

[20] For example, the Leofric Missal, the Missal of Robert Jumièges, and the Red Book of Darley. See further Thompson, *Dying*, 67–88; Kesling, *Medical Texts*, 88–91.

[21] *Bald's Leechbook I*, chs. 45, 47, 62–5, 88; *Bald's Leechbook II*, ch. 65; *Leechbook III*, chs. 41, 61–4, 67, 68, 71; *Lacnunga*, passim. All citations from the *Leechbooks* are taken from Cockayne, *Leechdoms*. *Bald's Leechbook I* and *II* and *Leechbook III* survive in London, British Library, Royal MS 12 D xvii. For those wishing to consult the original of any remedy cited, folio numbers are provided by Cockayne in the left-hand margin of his edition.

[22] Kesling, *Medical Texts*, 12, 182. Cf. a tradition in nineteenth- and early-twentieth-century scholarship assuming early medieval English doctors were uneducated, pagan 'wizards'; see, for example, Cockayne, *Leechdoms*, I:xxvii; Grattan and Singer, *Magic and Medicine*, 4–15; Storms, *Magic*; Rubin, *Medicine*, 13, 60–2; Talbot, *Medicine*, 10; Bonser, *Background*, 6–7. These ideas are no longer prevalent in scholarship on Old English medicine. For a recent overview and evaluation, see Trilling, 'Health'.

contain almost certainly required training and apprenticeship to be used correctly. The texts assume readers know how to identify, harvest, and preserve specific herbs; what amounts, measurements, and ratios one should use in preparing salves and tonics; how to distinguish between diseases; how to scarify, bloodlet, and cauterise; what equipment to use; how to apply prognostics and consult lunaria; and how to recite and perform multilingual rituals, including liturgical excerpts in Latin.[23] Physicians are often described as learned: the *Lacnunga* refers to *gelærede læceas* (educated physicians) and *afandad læcecræft* (proven medical practice), and describes naming diseases as the province of physicians.[24] *Bald's Leechbook* refers to tonics 'as doctors know how to make them' and suggests that the educated user should do both 'as you think good' and as the 'wisest' doctors teach.[25] The community of early medieval English physicians was probably small. *Bald's Leechbook* mentions two English physicians by name, Dun and Oxa, suggesting that the compendium was intended for the use of a select stratum of people who knew of one another, a medical community passing remedies between them.[26]

At the same time, however, most medical care in the early medieval period was probably carried out by practitioners with no knowledge of these elite medical texts. Patients were probably treated by secular clergy at isolated minster churches, community-based lay healers trained in apprenticeships with older local experts or simply through experience, and caregivers working within the home. Such practitioners leave little mark on the textual record, but must have existed. Numerous archaeological sites contain the graves of persons who experienced significant illness and impairment, but survived to adulthood and into old age – at least some of whom would have required and evidently received some form of care.[27] The prolific religious writer and scholar Ælfric, abbot of Cerne and Eynsham, repeatedly mentions the value of learned medicine in his homilies, but also insists that such practices must be distinguished from forbidden or illicit ones. This juxtaposition suggests that care from trained physicians competed with what Emily Kesling calls 'doctrinally unacceptable forms of healing'.[28]

Some of these practitioners were almost certainly women. Midwives likely existed in early medieval England as they did on the continent: the Junius manuscript, a magisterial codex of biblical poetry in Old English, contains

---

[23] van Arsdall, 'Medical Training', 430–2; Banham and Voth, 'Diagnosis', 171.

[24] *Lacnunga* nos. 75, 119, 120.

[25] van Arsdall, 'Medical Training', 432; *Bald's Leechbook I*, ch. 72; *Bald's Leechbook II*, ch. 18, passim.

[26] Banham, 'Dun', 61–70. [27] Lee, 'Disease', 713–15.

[28] Kesling, *Medical Texts*, 170. See Ælfric, 'Passion of St Bartholomew', esp. ll. 9–17, 244–334, and 'On Auguries' (ed. Skeat, *Lives of Saints*, 364–83).

three illustrations of mothers giving birth attended by other women.[29] Women probably also practiced medicine beyond obstetric care. Ælfric, in his homily 'On Auguries' (ll. 124–8), declares: 'ne sceal se cristena befrinan þa fulan wiccan be his gesundfulnysse, þeahðe heo secgan cunne sum ðincg þurh deofol' (the Christian man shall not ask the foul witch about his health, even though she is able to say something through [the power of] the devil). Penitentials and homilies mention women working with poisons, healing their children in evidently ritual modes, and providing abortions.[30] These texts collectively suggest that women did indeed practice medicine, including in ways that may have been considered unsanctioned, heterodox, or simply belonging to a more expansive definition of Christian devotion. The obstetric and gynaecological remedies preserved in the Old English medical texts are derived from classical sources, and if a popular feminine medical tradition existed, it has left few textual traces.[31] Yet the repeated association of women with medical care of children within the home and with reproductive expertise is telling. Indeed, nursing in individual homes and communities was probably one of the primary forms of medical care in the period, mentioned (albeit briefly) in several texts.[32]

The medieval hospital was generally an institution for the sick poor rather than a centre for medical intervention. It was also largely a post-Conquest innovation in Britain.[33] Certain early English burial sites – St John's Timberhill, for example, in which one-fifth of the graves contain individuals with leprosy advanced enough to be visible on the skeleton – have unusually high concentrations of persons with illnesses or physical differences that would likely have caused them impairment in life. Some archaeologists posit that these burial sites may have reflected the existence of an establishment providing nursing care nearby.[34] It is entirely possible, but by no means provable, that such establishments existed in England before the Conquest. Regardless, however, early medieval English medicine was mostly small-scale. Medical practice would have been centred around intimate interactions between patient and doctor – from a farmer consulting his minster priest, to a local midwife attending her neighbour's birth, to a king having his blood let by an abbot trained in France.

---

[29] Oxford, Bodleian Library, MS Junius 11, pp. 53, 62, 63.

[30] See Canons X16.02.01, B78.01.02, Y44.16.01 (Frantzen, 'Anglo-Saxon Penitentials'); for homiletic examples, see Ælfric, 'On Auguries', ll. 148–61, and 'Pentecost Octave' (ed. Pope, 415–47).

[31] On 'women's medicine', see most recently Voth, 'Women'; Sweany, 'Dangerous Voices'; Oswald, 'Courses'; Batten, 'Lazarus'.

[32] Alfred 17; Bede, *Historia ecclesiastica* IV.3; *Vita Dunstani* IV.2–3 (ed. Winterbottom and Lapidge, *Early Lives*). For discussion, see Dendle, *Demon Possession*, 88; Bolotina, 'Medicine and Society', 42, 63.

[33] See Orme and Webster, *English Hospital*.

[34] Roffey, 'Leper Hospitals', 210; Huggins, 'Excavation', 54–64.

Pathologies and Treatments

The archaeological record suggests that the people of early medieval England were generally well-nourished, with a substantial proportion of the population surviving into old age.[35] Illness, however, would have been common and often dangerous. The infant mortality rate was high, as was the percentage of women who died in childbirth or postpartum.[36] Burials and village archaeological sites reveal that intestinal parasites were more or less chronic, and osteoarthritic degeneration and other joint diseases occur frequently in excavated remains – unsurprising given the amount of regular physical labour completed by the average person.[37] Many skeletons also reveal signs of periostitis (inflammation of the connective tissue surrounding the bone), which can indicate a variety of different infections or stress injuries. Sinusitis, tuberculosis, leprosy, and dental diseases all appear fairly regularly in the archaeological record; several burials have also been documented of persons with cancer and poliomyelitis.[38] Diseases of the soft tissue leave no trace on the skeleton, but the medical manuscripts include numerous remedies for, among others, skin and eye ailments; fevers; pain in the head, ears, limbs, and joints; stomach and digestive tract ailments; coughs and lung diseases; internal pains in various locations; and boils, blains, and 'swellings' ranging from styes to haemorrhoids to tumours. A handful of surviving remedies address the starting and stopping of menstrual flow and the provision of obstetric care, but represent a small percentage of the medical corpus as a whole.[39] Other less quotidian sicknesses are also noted, including liver disease, paralysis, and necrosis of the flesh. Brief mentions are made of conditions that may be types of mental illness, such as *wedenheort* (*lit.* 'frenzied heart'), *ungemynd* (*lit.* 'un-mind', 'no mind'), *monaþseocnes* ('monthly-sickness', 'sickness at intervals', lunacy), and *gewitseocnes* (*lit.* sickness of the wits or sense), but in the absence of further details, we cannot be sure how these illnesses manifested in patients. Words for madness do gloss Latin terms referring to demonic possession, like *daemoniacus* and *energuminus*, and so it is possible that hagiographic descriptions of demonic possession provided a cultural explanation for certain kinds of mental illness, treated by ordained exorcists or clergy.[40] *Bræcseocnes* (breaking-sickness) and *fellseocnes* (falling-sickness), often grouped with mental illness words in glosses and medical texts, may have included symptoms we now understand as epilepsy or muscle control disorders. Though the *Anglo-Saxon Chronicle* mentions

---

[35] Lee, 'Disease', 706–8. Cf. Cameron, *Medicine*, 5–9.

[36] Sayer and Dickinson, 'Obstetric Death', 286–90.

[37] Thompson, *Dying*, 136; Lee, 'Disease', 707.   [38] Lee, 'Disease', 708–12.

[39] See Batten, 'Lazarus'; Voth, 'Women'.

[40] Dendle, *Demon Possession*, 93–4; Kesling, *Medical Texts*, 79, 84–5.

epidemic disease and the medical texts treat ailments that are undoubtedly signs of infection, all are too vaguely described to be parsed accurately, though we can be relatively certain that both influenza and ergotism were threats to the population.[41] The medical texts also feature illnesses whose names we cannot accurately translate, or which are difficult to map onto modern categories of disease – for example, the illness *þeor*, for which we have no satisfactory translation, or the relatively mysterious *ælf-adl* (elf-disease) or *feondes costunga* (temptations or trials of a demon).

The Old English medical texts are largely pharmaceutical, in that the vast majority of remedies they offer involve the creation of salves and poultices for external application, or tonic and emetic drinks for internal healing. Plants and herbs are by far the most important element in early medieval pharmacology, often blended with liquids like beer, wine, and water or with the products and parts of various animals, most commonly butter, gall, honey, and eggs.[42] This selection from the medical compendium *Bald's Leechbook* is typical:

> Wiþ heafod ece genim diles blostman, seoð on ele, smire þa þunwangan
> mid. Wiþ þon ilcan, genim heorotes hornes ahsan, meng wið eced ⁊ rosan
> seaw, bind on þæt wænge. Wiþ þon ilcan genim fæt ful grenre rudan leafa
> ⁊ senepes sædes cucler fulne, gegnid togædere, do æges þæt hwite to cucler
> fulne, þæt sio sealf sie þicce, smire mid feþere on þa healfe þe sar ne sie.[43]

> For head ache, take dill blossoms, seethe in oil, smear the temples with it.
> For the same, take ashes of hart's horn, mix with vinegar and rose juice,
> bind on the cheek. For the same, take a cup full of green rue leaves and
> a spoonful of mustard seeds, grind them together, add a spoon full of the
> white of an egg, so that the salve is thick, smear it with a feather on the
> side that is not sore.

A select few remedies include substances like spittle, blood, urine, breastmilk, and animal faeces. Some remedies also involve surgical procedures, though such techniques are mentioned far more rarely in the medical texts than the making of salves and drinks. Intentional amputation, trepanation, and the setting of broken bones are all attested in the archaeological record, and the texts also mention cautery, lancing, bloodletting, cupping, scarifying, and suturing.[44]

Plant names in Old English are famously hard to translate: how, for example, would we identify *attorlaþe* ('poison-loather'), which glosses betony, cockspur

---

[41] Horden, 'Millennium', 205.

[42] The text *Medicina de Quadrupedibus*, translated into Old English as part of the Herbarium Complex (discussed in the section 'Medical Texts in Early Medieval England'), contains exclusively remedies made with animal parts and products.

[43] *Bald's Leechbook*, ch. 1.

[44] Roberts and Cox, *Health*, 172, 216; Russcher and Bremmer, 'Fracture Treatment'; Banham and Voth, 'Diagnosis', 159.

grass, black nightshade, and other plants in Old English–Latin glossaries and whose appearance is never described in the medical texts?[45] Only a small proportion of names, like chervil and dill, are indisputably clear to us. Some, like crabapples, bindweeds, and berries, grew wild in England; others may have been cultivated in monastic gardens of the type tended by Ælfric Bata's *medicus*. Still others, like black pepper, could be obtained through what some sources suggest was a fairly robust spice trade with the continent.[46] Some remedies would have been relatively easy to make, involving native English herbs and inexpensive beer; others, as Bishop Cyneheard's plaintive letter reminds us, would have been all but impossible. Some Old English translations of Latin remedies swap out expensive or uncommon ingredients for more readily available ones: beer as an alternative to wine, oil of any kind (*ele*) instead of the labour-intensive rose oil (*oleum rosacium*) found so often in classical medicine.[47] Several pre-Conquest archaeological sites have turned up evidence of heavy use of plants that have some application as medical herbs or drugs, including – among many others – docks, nettle, elder, mayweed, bindweed, knotgrass, cinquefoils, self-heal, hemlock, nightshade, henbane, opium poppy, campions, various cresses and mints, meadowsweet, alliums, fennel, and hemp.[48] However, we do not know whether these plants were cultivated, imported, or gathered wild, and there are few cases of incontrovertible medical use.

A relatively small but notable percentage of the remedies in the Old English medical collections feature ritual elements apparently integral to their healing function. These include the recitation of prayers, masses, biblical quotations, and exorcistic formulae; the use of holy water, holy salt, and other church paraphernalia; spoken incantations in English, Latin, Greek, Hebrew, and Irish; written amulets; instructions to gather herbs in certain ways, visit certain locations, speak or keep silent, or make certain symbolic gestures; and the use of symbolically loaded ingredients, like the milk of a cow of one colour. A subset of these remedies are often designated in scholarship as 'charms': texts designed for performance that include a verbal (spoken or written) incantation, conjuration, or adjuration.[49] The difference between charm and prayer is often difficult to satisfactorily define – and a great number of indisputable prayers to God and his saints appear in the Old

---

[45] See Bierbaumer, *Wortschatz*. The extant illustrated copy of the Herbarium Complex contains schematic images. See D'Aronco, 'Plant Pharmacy', 135; Voigts, 'Plant Remedies', 252.

[46] Cameron, *Medicine*, 104; Voigts, 'Plant Remedies', 259–65.

[47] Kesling, *Medical Texts*, 144.   [48] Hall, 'Plant Life'; Moffett, 'Food Plants'.

[49] This definition is offered in Olsan, 'Inscription of Charms'. On the history of this term in scholarship – and on its many semantic difficulties – see Arthur, *'Charms'*, 8–17. As the title of Arthur's monograph suggests, however, the term 'charm' is hard to avoid as a shorthand for describing remedies that involve both incantatory speech and ritual action. I use Olsan's definition throughout the present study.

English medical texts. Charms and prayers both certainly belong to a paraliturgical 'penumbra' of texts used in early medieval England for practical devotion.[50] The prevalence of ritual remedies varies hugely by text: only seven to eight per cent of remedies in the hyper-scholarly *Bald's Leechbook*; eighteen per cent in the miscellany *Leechbook III*, which is especially interested in ailments caused by or related to non-human agents like demons; and twenty-seven per cent in the ecclesiastically influenced *Lacnunga*.[51] These remedies are rationally conceived within their early medieval cultural context, indistinguishable from other kinds of medicine within the Old English corpus, and cannot be dismissed as 'superstitious'.[52] The overlap between personal devotion and practical medicine was entirely sensible for medieval Christians, who considered the human body to be a microcosm of God's creation, medicinal healing a reestablishment of the divine order of a Christian universe, and pastoral care an essential aspect of clerical religious duty. The health of the body and the health of the soul are utterly interdependent, often conceptually inextricable, in these texts.[53] The ritual remedies included in the medical texts are heterogeneous and draw from many sources, but all contain Christian material; though they may not be entirely orthodox, they are unlikely to have been considered significantly heterodox.[54] Take, for example, a charm so popular it is occasionally referred to only by its first word, which appears in the *Lacnunga* in the following form:

> Sing ðis gebed on ða blacan blegene VIIII syðan; ærest Pater n(oste)r: Tigað tigað tigað calicet. aclu cluel sedes adclocles. acre earcre arnem. nonabiuð ær ærnem niðren arcum cunað arcum arctua fligara uflen binchi cuterii. nicuparam raf afð egal ufeln arta. arta. arta trauncula. trauncula; querite et inuenietis; adiuro te p(er) Patrem et Filium et Sp(iritu)m S(an)c(tu)m, non amplius crescas sed arescas. Sup(er) aspidem et basilliscum ambulabis et conculcabis leone(m) et draconem; crux Matheus, crux Marcus, crux Lucas, crux Iohannes.[55]

> Sing this prayer nine times on the black blains; before that the Our Father: '*Tigað tigað tigað calicet. aclu cluel sedes adclocles. acre earcre arnem. nonabiuð ær ærnem niðren arcum cunað arcum arctua fligara uflen binchi cuterii. nicuparam raf afð egal ufeln arta. arta. arta trauncula. trauncula*; seek and you shall find; I adjure you by the Father and Son and Holy Spirit, that you grow no further but dry up. Upon the asp and the basilisk you will walk and you will trample the lion and the dragon; cross Mathew, cross Mark, cross Luke, cross John.

---

[50] Liuzza, 'Prayers'.   [51] Meaney, 'Extra-Medical Elements', 47–54.
[52] See Paz, 'Magic'; Trilling, 'Health'.   [53] Trilling, 'Health', 67.
[54] Jolly, *Popular Religion*, 2–3; Gay, 'Incantations'. Old English texts distinguish between licit Christian incantations, prayers, and medical rituals, and forbidden incantations and rituals that do not draw upon the power of God; see, for example, Ælfric, 'Passion of St Bartholomew', ll. 319–25.
[55] *Lacnunga* no. 25.

The apparent 'nonsense' in this incantation includes multiple words and phrases in distorted Irish and possibly Hebrew, and is followed by Vulgate quotations from the Bible. The remedy also includes the phrase *adiuro te*, which appears in ecclesiastical exorcistic rites, and an evidently traditional rhyming phrase appearing in multiple medieval charms separated by geography and time (*non crescas sed arescas*).[56] The incantation as a whole is explicitly Christian, though it appears in no offices or books of prayer. It makes use of Latin as a sacred language, but also Irish – a language associated with religious learning in early medieval England – to create a commanding, otherworldly verbal performance. It may have been orally transmitted, given the garbling of the Irish words it contains, but in its recorded form it is intended for a literate practitioner with some facility with Latin and familiarity with ecclesiastical rites.

Looming over any discussion of early medieval medicine is a fundamentally unanswerable question: did these remedies work – and if so, how and for whom? Many ingredients listed in these texts have genuine medical properties: painkillers, antibiotics, anti-inflammatories, emmenagogues.[57] Scientific explorations have offered mixed results: one study found the remedies had no medical effect, whereas another found a *Leechbook* remedy for an eye infection to be effective against antibiotic-resistant MRSA.[58] We know so little about preparation that it is difficult to determine which, if any, remedies would have alleviated symptoms, though many elements involved – honey, alliums, gall, wine, copper salts – are in theory medically efficacious. We are also missing a key element of cultural context: the power of the placebo effect.[59] Modern scientific studies have consistently shown that if we believe we are receiving an efficacious treatment for certain ailments, our symptoms will improve. The performance of an incantation by a priest coupled with an herbal salve might well have alleviated the ailments of early medieval patients. The medical texts do not often discuss anatomy or aetiology, but they are constantly interested in the mitigation of symptoms: *him bið sona sel* (he will soon be better), the texts repeatedly promise.

More medicine survives in Old English than any other medieval vernacular: over sixty extant manuscripts contain medical information, from herbal remedies and charms to prognostics and bloodletting instructions, and the Old English medical collections constitute more than a thousand folios.[60] The dedication of

---

[56] Borsje, 'Éle', 204–5; Pettit, *Anglo-Saxon Remedies*, II: 22–6.

[57] Cameron, *Medicine*, 110–111, 120–123, 144.

[58] Brennessel, Drout, and Gravel, 'Reassessment'; Harrison et al., 'Antimicrobial Remedy'.

[59] See further Brackmann, 'Placebo'.

[60] Cameron, *Medicine*, 2. For a list of pre-Conquest manuscripts containing medical information, see Bolotina, 'Medicine and Society', 157–64.

so many expensive manuscript pages to medical writings, along with the addition of notes and new recipes to the collections and the modification of remedies for English ingredients, testifies to their immense cultural importance, and so any study of Old English medicine must address them in detail.

Medical Texts in Early Medieval England

Many of the remedies preserved in the pre-Conquest literary record are originally sourced from Latin texts that were the height of medical learning on the continent, while others have no known source and are presumably English in origin. Remedies travelled individually or in small groups, often abridged, recompiled, copied, and excerpted.[61] In addition to the four major Old English medical collections, small groups of remedies also appear in non-specialist manuscripts, including psalters, liturgical manuscripts, computistical treatises, and natural science texts. Examples include London, British Library, Cotton MS Caligula A xv, which contains extracts from Jerome and Isidore of Seville, numerous computus texts, and a collection of healing charms; Cambridge, Corpus Christi College MS 41, an edition of Bede's *Ecclesiastical History* in Old English whose margins contain medical remedies, a number of now-famous verse charms, and liturgical excerpts; and London, British Library, Cotton MS Vitellius E xviii, a psalter with a prefatory collection of remedies and prognostics.[62] Prayerbooks also often contain remedies – like London, British Library, Royal MS 2 A xx, featuring two groups of devotions for the cessation of menstrual bleeding (ff. 16 v, 49 r–v). These codices point to the close connection between spiritual and bodily health that animates many Old English texts.

It is often difficult to determine which Latin texts were available complete and which simply served as sources for translated remedies that circulated more or less independently. Texts that were available in their entirety in early medieval England prior to the mid-eleventh century include Pliny the Elder's *Naturalis historia*, Galen's *Ad Glauconem de methodo medendi*, the *Liber medicinalis* of Quintus Serenus Sammonicus, and possibly, given their prominence in the Old English medical collections, the Latin Alexander of Tralles, Oribasius's *Euporistes* and *Synopsis*, and the Galenic *Liber tertius*.[63] Sources for Old English remedies also include the other venerated Greek and Latin authors whose work was available on the continent: Vindicianus, Marcellus of Bordeaux, Philagrius of Epirus, Theodorus Priscianus, Caelius Aurelianus,

---

[61] Meaney, 'Versions', 237–50; Banham, 'Dun', 66; Kesling, *Medical Texts*, 4, 30.

[62] For example, Cotton Caligula A xv ff. 136r, 140r; Corpus Christi 41, pp. 182, 206–7, 350–3; Cotton Vitellius E xviii ff. 9r-15v. On these manuscripts, see Arthur, '*Charms*'; Jolly, 'Margins'; Pulsiano, 'Prefatory Material'.

[63] Kesling, *Medical Texts*, 20, 54–5.

Soranus of Ephesus, and Cassius Felix.[64] In the mid-eleventh century, major Galenic texts – including the Gariopontus-Petrocellus material that would soon anchor the curriculum of the Schola Salernitana – arrived in England.[65] Much of the Gariopontus-Petrocellus material was translated into the vernacular in the twelfth century, creating a text called the *Peri didaxeon*.

All translations of Latin remedies into Old English involve interpretation. The remedies are often edited, simplified, or stylistically altered, and many involve the synthesis of information from multiple sources.[66] Nowhere is the intellectual effort involved in such translation clearer than in the Herbarium Complex, a sizeable text (185 continuous chapters) that offers some of the most important Latin pharmaceutical treatises of the time translated into Old English: the herbal *De herba vettonica liber*; the popular fourth-century North African *Herbarius* of Pseudo-Apuleius; a selection of remedies from pseudo-Dioscorides's *Liber medicinae ex herbis femininis* and *Curae herbarum*; the pseudo-Apuleian *De taxone liber*; and the *Liber medicinae ex animalibus* attributed to Sextus Placitus Papiriensis, along with several chapters of unknown origin.[67] The translation was likely completed in the middle or second half of the tenth century and must have been a Benedictine Reform project undertaken by an experienced specialist at a major centre – Winchester, Canterbury, Worcester – and designed to create a comprehensive pharmaco-poeia in the vernacular.[68] The survival of four copies of the Herbarium Complex, dating from the late tenth to the twelfth centuries, testifies to its popularity.[69]

Older than the Herbarium Complex is the medical compendium referred to as *Bald's Leechbook* (London, British Library, Royal MS 12 D xvii). Consisting of more than one hundred folios of medical remedies drawn largely from major Latin sources (the *Physica Plinii*; the *Liber tertius*; Marcellus; Alexander; Oribasius), *Bald's Leechbook* seems to have been made for a user called Bald by a scribe called Cild, according to a Latin colophon in the text.[70] Like the Herbarium Complex, the *Leechbook* was a massive intellectual undertaking, but in this case the compiler gathered and sorted remedies that were already circulating pre-translated into English, and also translated new remedies

---

[64] Cameron, 'Medical Knowledge', 134–48; Doyle, 'Medicine'.

[65] Banham, 'Mainstream', 345.　　[66] Kesling, *Medical Texts*, 36, 39, 133–40.

[67] The section of the Complex that offers remedies made from animal parts is usually referred to as the *Medicina de Quadrupedibus*.

[68] Kesling, *Medical Texts*, 147–52.

[69] London, British Library, Cotton MS Vitellius C iii; Oxford, Bodleian Library, MS Hatton 76; London, British Library, Harley MS 585; London, British Library, Harley MS 6258B. Edition in Niles and D'Aronco, *Medical Writings*. See further Garner, *Hybrid Healing*, 160–94.

[70] Cameron, 'Sources and Their Use', 154–5, 166; Talbot, *Medicine*, 19.

specifically for the compilation.[71] The text is divided into two books: Book I begins by offering remedies in head-to-foot order, and then switches to remedies grouped by disease, while Book II describes different internal organs one by one and lists remedies for ailments associated with them, including some passages on medical theory. The Royal manuscript was copied at Winchester in the mid-tenth century, by the same scribe who copied the entries for 925–955 CE in the Parker manuscript of the *Anglo-Saxon Chronicle*.[72] The collection itself, however, was likely compiled for Bald in the late ninth century, probably also at Winchester, making it part of the program of written vernacular knowledge spearheaded by King Alfred, in his reign-defining efforts to make Latin learning accessible to an English-speaking population.[73] Indeed, several remedies in *Bald's Leechbook* claim to have been sent to Alfred by the Patriarch of Jerusalem,[74] firmly associating either the original compilation or the Royal copy with Alfred, the court of Wessex, and the vernacular renaissance of the ninth century.

Following *Bald's Leechbook* in the Royal manuscript is an eighteen-folio medical miscellany copied by the same scribe, referred to as *Leechbook III*.[75] The remedies are in a much looser head-to-toe order, and the text is less comprehensive and features almost no medical theory. It has the smallest percentage of remedies with identifiable Latin sources and a particularly large percentage of remedies containing only native ingredients and using exclusively English plant names.[76] It also contains a particular concentration of remedies for illnesses ascribed to anthropomorphic agents, including elves, demons, and *nihtgengan* (night-walkers), discussed in the following section.

The fourth major Old English medical collection is a miscellany without a table of contents or clear organising scheme, given the scholarly title *Lacnunga*. It is preserved in London, British Library, Harley MS 585, alongside the Herbarium Complex. *Lacnunga* was compiled in the late tenth or early eleventh century, potentially at Winchester, and shares a number of short remedies with both *Bald's Leechbook* and *Leechbook III*.[77] The overlap suggests the compiler(s) drew on the same body of pre-translated remedies circulating individually and in small groups that furnished the other medical compendia. Some scholars describe *Lacnunga* as a commonplace book or working notebook for a physician, but parchment was expensive and the copying in the manuscript itself is clean, making it more likely to have been a compilation of all the available medical material gathered in a particular

---

[71] Kesling, *Medical Texts*, 28–30.   [72] Wright, *Bald's Leechbook*, 11–22.

[73] Banham, 'Millennium', 232; Meaney, 'Versions', 251.   [74] *Bald's Leechbook II*, ch. 64.

[75] Wright, *Bald's Leechbook*, 14; Meaney, 'Versions', 237.   [76] Kesling, *Medical Texts*, 58–9.

[77] Kesling, *Medical Texts*, 96; Banham, 'Millennium', 232; Meaney, 'Versions', 257–64.

scriptorium, written down without discarding or sorting.[78] Scholars have also characterised *Lacnunga* as particularly interested in folklore and exotica.[79] *Lacnunga* does have a high percentage of remedies involving ritual, but they are overwhelmingly ecclesiastical in nature, clearly made by and for literate users, with significant liturgical elements. The collection contains remedies with notable parallels in Old English liturgical and ecclesiastical manuscripts – prayers, litanies, biblical quotations, and selections from the mass and the Divine Office – and remedies that also appear in major devotional texts, including the *Book of Cerne* and the *Book of Nunnaminster*. The compiler seems to have been particularly interested in remedies that assert the power of language, including Latin prayers, Greek and Hebrew phrases, and a significant percentage of the surviving incantations that contain recognisable Old English verse.[80] These charms, like the remedies in *Leechbook III*, often attribute disease to a range of supernatural beings, including elves, dwarves (*dweorges*), night-walkers, and witches – perfectly compatible with a Christian world view, though culturally specific to early medieval England.[81]

These brief mentions of malevolent supernatural creatures, however, raise a new set of questions: who are these agents of disease? How does this idea of illness fit in with remedies that have sources in classical texts adhering to humoral theory? How did the early medieval English think about health and sickness? The answers to these questions offer new insights into early medieval understandings of the body, the supernatural, and the place of humankind in the postlapsarian Christian cosmos – and so it is to metaphors of illness that this study now turns.

Sickness and the Body

Different sociocultural communities use a wide variety of models to explain how disease works, and therefore how the sick body can be safeguarded and returned to health. Anthropologist Nigel Barley notes that there are three major ways of thinking about sickness:

> Disease can be seen as caused by the invasion of the body by alien matter or a force from without. Treatment then consists in removing it. It can be

---

[78] Cameron, *Medicine*, 34; Banham, 'Dun', 60; cf. Meaney, 'Practice', 232.

[79] Dendle, *Demon Possession*, 89; Cameron, *Medicine*, 34; Talbot, *Medicine*, 22; Rubin, *Medicine*, 60–2; Grattan and Singer, *Magic and Medicine*, 7, 15.

[80] Kesling, *Medical Texts*, 96–103.

[81] The word 'supernatural' did not enter the English language until the fifteenth century. It is useful here for describing powerful non-human, non-animal beings and forces thought to transcend the laws of perceptible physical reality. In early medieval English literature, creatures we would consider to be 'supernatural' are treated as part of a hostile natural world. See Neville, *Representations*, 2–6.

viewed as the loss, by a man, of something normally inherent to him. In this case, treatment consists in returning it to him. A third possible view would be to see disease as caused by a disruption of natural order within the body. Here, treatment would entail re-establishing that order.[82]

The Old English medical texts often seem uninterested in disease aetiology. The majority of remedies do not describe the causes of a particular illness but simply address the symptom they intend to cure – a headache, knee pain, swollen eyes, skin lesions – or name the function of the tonic or emollient they describe – a lung-salve, a *spiwdrenc* (emetic). Their primary concern is the amelioration of suffering. A representative recipe for a salve reads as follows:

> To wensealfe: nim elenan ⁊ cyrfillan ⁊ hræmnes fot, Ængliscne næp ⁊ finul ⁊ saluian ⁊ suþernewuda, ⁊ cnuca tosomne, ⁊ nim garleaces godne dæl; cnuca, ⁊ wring þurh cla\u00f0 on gemered hunig; þonne hit swi\u00f0e gesoden sy, þonne do \u00f0u pipor ⁊ sideware, gallengar ⁊ gingifre ⁊ rinde ⁊ lawerbergean ⁊ pyretran, godne dæl ælces be \u00f0ære mæ\u00f0e, ⁊ sy\u00f0\u00f0an hit swa gemænged þara wyrta wos ⁊ þæt hunig, þonne seo\u00f0 \u00f0u hit twa swa swi\u00f0e swa hit ær wæs; þonne hæfs þu gode sealfe wi\u00f0 wennas ⁊ wi\u00f0 nyrwet.[83]

> For a wen-salve: take elecampane and chervil and *hræmnes* foot, English rape and fennel and sage and southernwood, and pound together, and take a good portion of garlic; pound, and wring through a cloth into purified honey; when it is thoroughly boiled, then add pepper and zedoary, galingale and ginger and [cinnamon] bark and laurel-berries and feverfew, a good portion of each according to the strength, and after the juice of the plants and the honey has been mixed thus, then boil it twice as strongly as it was before; then you will have a good salve for wens and for shortness of breath.

Wenn is a word used to describe cutaneous swellings (cysts, boils, tumours) as well as chest oppression – hence, perhaps, the relationship between *wennas* and *nyrwet* (shortness of breath).[84] Chest oppression may have been understood to be a kind of internal swelling, as there can apparently be 'wennas æt mannes heortan' (wens at a person's heart).[85] This semantic linking of 'internal' and 'external' illnesses suggests that the cutaneous swellings designated by the term *wenn* were not considered to reside on the surface of the body, but underneath it. The same illness can be deep within the flesh or just below its defining outer bounds. As in the vast majority of other Old English remedies, the symptoms –

---

[82] Barley, 'Magico-Medicine', 68.   [83] *Lacnunga* no. 30.
[84] *Leechbook I*, ch. 2; *Leechbook III*, chs. 30–32, 59; *Lacnunga* nos. 30, 72, 82, 112, 176. See also London, British Library, Cotton MS Domitian A.i f. 55v; London, Wellcome Historical Medical Library, MS 46 f. 144r.
[85] *Lacnunga* no. 82.

wennas and *nyrwet* – are presented on their own, isolated from the context of the rest of the body. This localisation of the ailment or dysfunction suggests the idea of a body that is otherwise and by its nature free of sickness, or which by nature functions in a certain way, until individual problems located in specific body parts arise and must be individually corrected through the application of the corresponding remedy. The physician creates the salve from a variety of plants, which must be correctly processed, employed in concert with one another, and evaluated for their individual *mæð* (measure of power). The Old English medical corpus elsewhere ascribes *mægen* (might, strength) to plants and in a number of remedies treats plants themselves as agents with will, intention, and a capacity for both capriciousness and danger.[86] The correct, multi-stage processing of the plants transforms this natural, and perhaps ambivalent, power into a positive instrument of the physician's science with the ability to diminish or erase symptoms: a *gode sealfe* (good salve). *God* seems to be multivalent here, likely indicating efficaciousness, value, and the capacity to enact a moral good – the healing of the sick.

Only a relatively small percentage of remedies ascribe illness to a cause; most, like the wen salve recipe, treat the patient's symptoms as their own cause. When medical remedies do assert that disease is produced by a specific mechanism, therefore, it is both interesting and notable that they refer most often to anthropomorphised supernatural agents, creatures who seek to break open and invade the body. The individual patient's experience of illness is elevated into a struggle against hostile forces in a postlapsarian world, a microcosmic battlefield reflecting the macrocosmic dynamics of the medieval Christian universe. Remedies with ritual elements more frequently identify an agent of disease causation than those without such elements, suggesting the possibility that different kinds of medicine apply to different illnesses (or assessments of those illnesses by the physician in question). Yet this 'invasive model' of disease is of a piece with the remedy already discussed, which assumes the body is afflicted with an anomalous symptom that must be removed from, or undone within, otherwise healthy flesh. Other learned models of the sick body appear in the surviving corpus – Bede, for example, cites changes in the air as a cause of epidemic disease,[87] and the medical texts engage with humoral theory in subtle and unusual ways, as discussed in the following – but consistent reassertions of the metaphor of disease as invader in the medical texts and in numerous Old English literary texts point to its cultural importance, and

---

[86] Fay, 'Farmacy'.

[87] Bede, *De natura rerum* (trans. Kendall and Wallis), 154–5. A similar statement appears in biblical commentary; see 'Supplementary Commentary on Genesis, Exodus, and the Gospels', 28, in Bischoff and Lapidge, *Biblical Commentaries*, 394.

reveal a preoccupation with policing the boundaries of the body, shoring up its points of entry against incursion, and maintaining the self as an invulnerable, inviolate whole.

Humoral Theory in Early Medieval English Medicine

Humoral theory is arguably the most widespread model of the human body and its various ailments found in the literature of the European Middle Ages. The humoral model is derived from the works of Galen of Pergamon, a Greek physician and philosopher active in the second century, whose writings dominated medieval understandings of medicine. Humoral theory posits that the body contains four humours: blood, red or yellow bile, black bile, and phlegm, which each possess a different combination of heat or cold with moisture or dryness – red bile, for example, is hot and dry, while blood is hot and moist. The humours must exist in balanced proportions in the body for optimum health, and an excess of any given humour causes sickness, as well as changes in the patient's emotional state. Humoral excess is corrected by the ingestion of medicines with opposite properties (cold for heat, moisture for dryness, etc.) as well as bloodletting, scarification, cupping, and induced vomiting, which purportedly drain humours physically from the patient.

Latin medical texts available in early medieval England, and Latin source remedies for a great number of Old English medical texts, implicitly rely upon humoral theory, and some articulate that theory explicitly. The humoral model of the body was certainly known in early medieval England as early as the eighth century. Bede discusses the four humours – though he does not mention their role in medicine – in his *De temporum ratione*, presumably drawing on both the *Epistola Vindiciani*, a medical treatise that circulated in whole or in part in early medieval England, and Isidore of Seville's *Etymologiae*, a highly influential and popular etymological encyclopaedia that circulated extensively in medieval Europe and includes a medical treatise drawing on the works of Caelius Aurelianus.[88] Humoral theory persisted in scientific treatises written by educated, Latin-literate authors: the *Enchiridion*, a scientific manual written by the monk Byrhtferth of Ramsey (c.1011), names the four humours in Latin and associates them with the four elements (air, fire, earth, and water), while the twelfth-century medical treatise *Peri didaxeon* directly translates a passage on the humours from the *Petrocellus Tereoperica*, noting that there are four humours (*feower wætun*) named as *blod*, *swerta gealle*, *ruwa gealle*, and *wæte*.[89] A number of pre-Conquest Old English

---

[88] Bede, *De temporum ratione* (trans. Wallis), 100–2.

[89] Byrhtferth of Ramsey, *Enchiridion* (ed. Baker and Lapidge, 10–12); *Peri didaxeon*, ch. 1 (ed. Niles and D'Aronco, *Medical Writings*, 534).

medical or medical-adjacent codices include instructions for bloodletting, a methodology inherently indebted to humoral theory. In the four major pre-Conquest texts of the Old English medical corpus – the *Herbarium* complex, *Bald's Leechbook*, *Leechbook III*, and the *Lacnunga* – a handful of remedies note that illnesses can be generated by excessive heat, cold, moisture, or dryness, and that the remedies change accordingly for each cause, along with several mentions of fluids in the body that can be either hot or cold.[90] The majority of these references appear in *Bald's Leechbook II*, which largely deals with internal medicine and has theoretical ambitions not shared by other Old English medical texts; *Leechbook III*, by contrast, which contains the highest percentage of English remedies without Latin sources, does not mention humoral theory at all.[91] Some scholars take these references collectively to mean that early medieval English physicians universally understood imbalances of the four natural humours to be the foremost cause of diseases in their patients.[92]

The Old English medical texts as a whole, however, arguably do not show a high level of engagement with the fullness of humoral theory as detailed in their Latin source texts. Instead, they seem to adhere to an altered, adjusted model of the role of bodily fluids in disease causation. The four pre-Conquest medical compilations contain no texts or remedies that articulate the central tenets of the humoral model. Even Old English bloodletting texts, and remedies that mention hot and cold sources for illness, do not discuss the humours, and indeed no pre-Conquest Old English medical text acknowledges that they are four distinct substances.[93] The Old English translation of Boethius's *De consolatione philosophiae*, an immensely popular text in early medieval Europe, in fact removes Galenic humoral metaphors present in the original, suggesting that such metaphors were considered either incomprehensible or unimportant by the translator(s).[94] It is telling that neither Bede nor Byrhtferth names the four humours in the vernacular or addresses their medical functions in any detail, because the pre-Conquest Old English medical texts essentially lack a humoral vocabulary. Old English remedies discussing bodily fluids universally use the word *wæta*, which can apparently refer to humours but simply means 'moisture, fluid' and can refer not only to any 'humour' but also to pus, mucus, liquids for drinking, or any kind of wetness.[95] Translations of Latin remedies that mention humours refer only to *wætan*, not to phlegm or black bile. Very occasionally the medical texts use the difficult word *oman*, which might refer to red bile but is

---

[90] For example, *Bald's Leechbook I*, ch. 1; *Bald's Leechbook II*, chs. 27, 28, 36; *Lacnunga* no. 173.

[91] Kesling, *Medical Texts*, 55–57.   [92] E.g., Bonser, *Background*, 36; Doyle, 'Medicine', 121.

[93] Ayoub, 'Old English *Wæta*', 341–6; Meaney, 'Practice', 224; Banham, 'Millennium', 234–6.

[94] Sweany, 'Imagination', 15. See *Old English Boethius* (ed. Godden and Irvine), 1:51, 61–68.

[95] *Bosworth-Toller Anglo-Saxon Dictionary* s.v. 'Wæta'; Doyle, 'Medicine', 124, 144, 178, 186.

also used of skin ailments like erysipelas.[96] A single *Bald's Leechbook* remedy refers to 'þæs geallancoðe þa readan' (this red 'gealle' disease), but it is unclear whether the word *gealle* here means 'bile' in the humoral sense or refers instead to a raised sore.[97] The same chapter goes on to say that 'þa hwitan lichoman beoð mearuwran ⁊ tedran þonne þa blacan ⁊ þa readan' (the white bodies/fleshes are softer and weaker than the black and the red), which could refer to bodies in which a given humour predominates, but the preceding remedy consistently uses 'black' (*sweart, blac*) – and possibly also 'red' (*read*), in this context – to describe the literal colour of diseased flesh.[98] The description of bodily fluids with medical words that have other unrelated meanings, as well as a general refusal to distinguish bodily fluids from one another, indicates that knowledge of the identities and functions of the four humours likely was not considered universally essential to the medical practice documented in the Old English textual corpus.

More importantly, the Old English translations of remedies that refer to the humours do not ascribe disease to the imbalance of naturally occurring bodily substances, but to the presence of *yfelan wætan* (evil fluids) in the body, which must be done away with (*don aweg*), healed (*lacnian*), drawn out (*ateon ut*), driven out and diminished (*todrifð ond lytlað*), or cleansed (*cleansian*) from the flesh.[99] These fluids are described as poisonous and treated as venoms to be extracted; they are disease agents in and of themselves, evil substances that must be purged from the patient. One *Bald's Leechbook* remedy is simply a set of instructions for 'ðu man sceal þa wætan ond þa wonsceaftan utan lacnian' (how one may heal fluids and misery) with a salve, treating the presence of bodily fluids themselves as a disease symptom and the cause of the patient's distress.[100] These remedies work to accommodate the humoral theory of their Latin source material – describing 'evil' bodily humours as the cause of disease, acknowledging the importance of distinguishing between hot and cold ailments – without necessarily including or drawing upon its fundamental model of disease causation, that of imbalance between four distinct, naturally occurring bodily elements. English translators of Latin medical material were willing to alter their sources where important or convenient, making such adjustments as removing a reference to the spirit (Latin *anima*) residing in the liver because

---

[96] Ayoub, 'Old English *Wæta*', 341–2. For an example of ambiguous use of *oman*, see *Bald's Leechbook I*, ch. 39. *Peri didaxeon*, the only text to translate the names of the humours into the vernacular, uses *oman* immediately afterwards to mean erysipelas (ch. 2).

[97] *Bald's Leechbook I*, ch. 35. See *Dictionary of Old English A to I* s.v. 'Gealle'.

[98] *Bald's Leechbook I*, ch. 35.

[99] *Bald's Leechbook I*, chs. 1, 35; *Bald's Leechbook II*, chs. 1, 25, 27–30, 38, 42, 59. See Cameron, 'Bald's Leechbook', 12; Meaney, 'View', 14.

[100] *Bald's Leechbook II*, ch. 38.

early medieval English models of the body elsewhere attested locate the spirit in the heart.[101] Such changes are not a sign of misunderstanding but of intellectual and cultural reinterpretation. The simplified, looser version of humoral theory targets evil fluids within otherwise healthy flesh, much in the way the wen-salve remedy treats swellings as isolated anomalies to be targeted for correction. While Old English iterations of Latin remedies retain a number of humoral principles – bloodletting and emetics work to purge the body of undesirable substances, altering its internal function – they distinguish the fluids of illness from the substances of the patient's normally functioning flesh and treat them instead as invaders or poisons. Such an interpretation brings the Latin source material conceptually in line with the most prominent model of disease aetiology found in the Old English medical texts, insofar as they address causation: illness as incursive agent.

Agents of Disease

When Old English medical remedies refer to the causes of disease, they most frequently use an external–internal model: the body is entered from without by alien matter or forces, often described as adversarial, mobile entities usually possessing some kind of volition or intent.[102] *Wyrmas* (worms) are mentioned over a hundred and fifty times as the cause of ailments in the medical texts, including *inwyrmas* (inward-moving worms) and *smeawyrmas* (creeping or penetrating worms), described as eating flesh and growing inside patients.[103] The word *wyrm* is a multivalent term that presumably refers to any number of parasites in a medical context, and Old English remedies treat worms in all parts of the body, from the eyes to the innards to the feet. In literary and religious texts, worms are persistently linked to mortality, decay, disease, and the consumption of the human body, featuring prominently in descriptions of Hell. Indeed, medical descriptions of penetrating worms eating flesh recall the images in Old English poetry and homiletic prose of corpses consumed by *wyrmas* who bore through eyes, crack open heads, and chew holes in necks – where the imagery is of being entered, laid (burst, split, torn) open, and exposed.[104] Poison (*attor*) is another frequently named cause of disease.[105] Remedies for *attor* do not merely seek to counteract harmful ingested substances. Rather, 'poisons' are

---

[101] Kesling, *Medical Texts*, 41.

[102] Barley, 'Magico-Medicine', 68; Künzel, 'Concepts', 245–56; Sweany, 'Imagination', 23, 31–2, 49; Thompson, *Dying*, 132.

[103] For all instances of *wyrm* in the medical corpus, see *Dictionary of Old English Corpus*, Simple Search, Cameron Number B21/B23, 'Wyrm'. See further Ogura, 'OE *Wyrm*'.

[104] For example, *Soul and Body I* ll. 119–24. For further discussion, see Thompson, *Dying*, 117–51.

[105] See *Dictionary of Old English Corpus*, Simple Search, Cameron Number B21/B23, 'Attor', 'Attr-', 'Atr-'.

several times described as flying venoms (*fleogende attor*) that move through the air seeking out human flesh, and may be a metaphor for infectious disease.[106] They thus demonstrate a kind of hostile intent, and in one verse charm, they are also conflated with 'þam laþan þe geond lond færeð' (the loathsome one that travels throughout the land),[107] a personified disease agent that, like these 'flying poisons', seems to originate in undomesticated spaces, to move pervasively through the landscape, and to breach the defences of the flesh. These disease agents may represent real observations of illness – intestinal parasites, the spread of symptoms between persons – but also reveal essential cultural concerns explicitly present in a subset of the Old English medical writings. Illnesses emerge from a hostile natural world. They are fundamentally opposed to humanity, and in some cases aligned with the demonic. The human body is evidently fragile, subject to constant menaces, and vulnerable to being entered, broken open, or consumed.

Indeed, a number of Old English medical remedies also refer to supernatural, anthropomorphised disease agents. A number of illnesses are attributed or some-how related to beings called *ylfe* (sing. *ælf*), a term usually translated by its modern descendant 'elves'.[108] We know very little about early medieval elves, though they also appear in Old Norse and Middle High German texts.[109] They are likely humanoid supernatural beings, associated with brightness and beauty in certain texts but closely linked to demons in the majority of the corpus.[110] Elf-related illnesses, including *ælfadl* (elf-sickness), *ælfsiden* (elvish influence), and *ælfsogoða* (elf-related internal pain) appear across the Old English medical corpus.[111] Elves are consistently linked to spasmic and delirious symptoms, including epilepsy; internal pains; and sores or wounds on the skin.[112] Elves are named as one possible agent among several who can cause the ailment *gescot* ('shot', i.e. internal pain) – including in a verse charm that equates *gescot* with sudden, severe pain caused by an invisible spear shot by elves, witches, or (possibly) non-Christian gods.[113] Internal pains and skin wounds may well be linked to elves because both were understood to be caused by this sort of projectile intrusion, evidence that the patient had been 'stabbed', assaulted, or penetrated. A greater number of illnesses are attributed to the malevolent influence of demons (*deofles* or *feondas*). Demon-caused ailments, like the elf-related

---

[106] *Bald's Leechbook II*, chs. 45, 64; *Lacnunga* nos. 17, 76, 126.   [107] *Lacnunga* no. 76.

[108] For example, *Leechbook I*, ch. 64; *Leechbook II*, ch. 65; *Leechbook III*, chs. 41, 54, 61–3; *Lacnunga* 29, 127.

[109] See Hall, *Elves*, 98, 108 125–6; Ármann Jakobsson, 'Beware'.

[110] See further Hall, *Elves*; Thun, 'Elves'; Jolly, *Popular Religion*.

[111] On *ælfsogoða*, see Hall, 'Calling the Shots', 204.

[112] Jolly, *Popular Religion*, 133; see remedies cited in note 108.

[113] Hall, 'Calling the Shots', 200; *Bald's Leechbook II*, ch. 65; *Lacnunga* no. 127.

illnesses mentioned earlier, are generally grouped with remedies for mind-altering and convulsive afflictions.[114] While the medical texts do not mention the kind of indwelling or manipulative possession found in saints' lives, demonic influence on, access to, and injury or invasion of the body seems to be a relevant concern.[115] The ailment referred to as *feondseocnes* and *deofolseocnes* (fiend- or devil-sickness), for example, is defined in *Bald's Leechbook* as 'þonne deofol þone monnan fede oððe hine inan gewealde mid adle' (when a devil nourishes a man or controls him within with disease).[116] The *Old English Herbarium* equates devil-sickness with *gewitleaste* (madness, senselessness)[117] and the word elsewhere glosses *daemoniacus*, suggesting that the ailment was understood on some level to be a displacement of the patient from control of their own body. The *Lacnunga* also contains three remedies against a *dweorh*, a term usually translated by its modern descendant 'dwarf', which seems to refer to both a supernatural creature and a dangerously high fever.[118] Like elves, dwarves as supernatural beings are mentioned in Old Norse texts, but we know little about them in an English context other than that they were probably thought to be humanoid and small. A lead amulet found in Norfolk dating to anywhere between the eighth and eleventh centuries bears the inscription *Dead is dwerg* (the dwarf is dead) above a drawing of a face in profile, and the word glosses Latin terms for semi-mythical small peoples across the early medieval period.[119]

The remedies for these sicknesses consistently make use of exorcistic elements, liturgical prayers, ecclesiastical *materia medica*, and adjurations or commands that a hostile being be expelled from the patient. This textual evidence suggests that names like 'elf-sickness' or 'devil-sickness' are not fossilisations but rituals intended to combat 'real' anthropomorphised disease creatures. Several remedies speak explicitly about the reality of such supernatural beings: a *Leechbook* remedy for 'feondes costunge' (the trials, temptations, or afflictions of a demon) encourages the patient to put herbs under their pillow and over their door 'ne mæg þe deofol sceþþan inne ne ute' (so the devil cannot hurt you within or without), while a remedy copied a few folios later for *ælfadl* warns the physician that they may encounter 'hwæthwega egeslices' (something terrifying) during the ritualised gathering of elecampane to treat the patient.[120] Even if these

---

[114] See, for example, *Leechbook I*, ch. 63; *Leechbook II*, chs. 65–6; *Leechbook III*, chs. 2, 12, 41, 58, 61–2, 64, 67; *Lacnunga* nos. 29, 65, 170.

[115] Dendle, *Demon Possession*, 143–4, 151.   [116] *Leechbook I*, ch. 63.

[117] *Old English Herbarium* (ed. de Vriend), ch. 132.4.

[118] *Dictionary of Old English A to I* s.v. 'Dweorg'; Meaney, 'View', 19; Pettit, *Lacnunga*, II:174.

[119] On the inscription, see Hines, 'Runic Literacy ', and entry NMS-63179C under the Portable Antiquities Scheme (https://finds.org.uk/database/artefacts/record/id/751600). For glosses, see *Dictionary of Old English A to I* s.v. 'Dweorg'.

[120] *Leechbook III*, chs. 58, 62.

disease names and disease-banishing rituals are metaphorical rather than literal, however, they reflect an understanding of illness as external, incursive, and malicious.

This model of the body is in no way incompatible with the humoral theory that informs the Latin medical texts available in pre-Conquest England and appears in a somewhat altered form in *Bald's Leechbook* and *Lacnunga*. Both models see the ideal, healthy body as a closed system capable of self-regulation. Both models also propose to mediate and rehabilitate the imperfect reality of the body as a dangerously porous entity, susceptible to outside influence that can cause internal disruption or imbalance, but also capable of adjusting in response to environmental changes. Remedies that adhere to the incursive model – ascribing disease to demonic agents or using religious language and materials to remove malign influence – see the solution to be the extraction and removal of the dangerous agent, followed by a shoring-up of the body's defences. Remedies that are informed by the humoral model or its modified English iteration use the porousness of the body to their advantage, introducing curative substances to help the body right itself or counteract the presence or excess of a dangerous substance. Both models are interested in purgation: exorcism, banishment, spitting, blowing, bloodletting, induced vomiting. The true vulnerability – and potential – of the body, in the early medieval English medical understanding, is its ability to act as a site of interchange between self and other, inside and outside, individual and surrounding world.

Bodily Metaphors in Early Medieval English Medicine

Remedies that attribute sickness to demonic influence, elvish assaults, and the insidious creeping of worms reveal a specific, persistent anxiety in the Old English medical texts: a concern with the violent and intentional breaking-open of the body through intimate contact with the inhuman other. Illness is treated as a breach or violation, and many of these remedies seek to treat the ailment in question by expelling or banishing the antagonistic agent and restoring the body to wholeness. Sickness is fundamentally an exchange of power. To be diseased is to surrender agency, to submit to or be violently overcome by a malevolent force.

Remedies that adhere to this model of illness use a variety of images and metaphors, and employ specific language, to describe and address these boundary violations. Liturgical quotation and ecclesiastical *materia medica* counteract and banish demonic or elvish influence. Poison, too, can be drawn out through Christian ritual, as in one multilingual remedy that asks God to destroy the venom within the patient's body.[121] Not infrequently, however, the metaphors are martial. 'Penetrating' worms are removed from the body by a garbled Irish incantation that begins *Gonomil orgomil marbumil* (roughly: I wound the beast, I hit the beast, I kill the beast).[122] A long charm against flying poisons and the 'loathsome one that travels throughout the land' calls upon nine plants, some of which are poisonous or inedible themselves, to 'stand against' (*wiðstandan*), 'crash against' (*wiðstunan*), 'put to flight' (*fleon*), and 'drive out' (*wrecan, weorpan*) the venoms that the charmer eventually blows out of the patient (*of ðe geblawe*) to banish them from the flesh.[123] Another medical incantation found in *Leechbook III* intended to treat chickenpox or a similar skin ailment addresses the patient's lesions as battle wounds. The incantation begins: 'Ic benne awrat betest beadowræda', which may be translated as either 'I have written out for the wounds the best of battle troops' – perhaps referring to the names of the plants used in the accompanying herbal remedy – or 'I have bound around the wounds the best of battle bandages' – perhaps referring to either literal dressings or to the incantation's magical action designed to seal off and close up the sores.[124] The tools of the healer are transformed into the tools of war, and the blisters of chickenpox are transformed into injuries sustained in conflict with an armed enemy. The illness, unsurprisingly, is named as *wæterælfadl* (watery elf-disease).

Wið færstice ('against a sudden, stabbing pain'), the aforementioned charm for *gescot*, sees disease as a consequence of a battlefield defeat:

> Hlude wæran hy, la hlude,   ða hy ofer þone hlæw ridan,
> wæran anmode   ða hy ofer land ridan.
> Scyld ðu ðe nu, þu ðysne nið   genesan mote!
> Ut, lytel spere,   gif herinne sie!
> Stod under linde,   under leohtum scylde,
> þær ða mihtigan wif   hyra mægen beræddon,
> ⁊ hy gyllende   garas sændan.
> Ic him oðerne   eft wille sændan,
> fleogende flane   forane togeanes.
> Ut lytel spere,   gif hit herinne sy! . . .
> Gif herinne sy   isenes dæl,
> hægtessan geweorc,   hit sceal gemyltan.
> Gif ðu wære on fell scoten,   oððe wære on flæsc scoten,
> oððe wære on blod scoten,
> oððe wære on lið scoten,   næfre ne sy ðin lif atæsed.
> Gif hit wære esa gescot   oððe hit wære ylfa gescot
> oððe hit wære hægtessan gescot   nu ic wille ðin helpan.
> Þis ðe to bote esa gescotes,   ðis ðe to bote ylfa gescotes,

---

[121] *Lacnunga* no. 64.   [122] *Lacnunga* nos. 26, 27.   [123] *Lacnunga* no. 76.
[124] *Leechbook III*, ch. 63. See *Dictionary of Old English A to I* s.v. 'Beadowræda'.

ðis ðe to bote hægtessan gescotes;   ic ðin wille helpan.
Fled þær   on fyrgenhæfde.
Hal westu!   Helpe ðin drihten.[125]

(Loud were they, lo, loud, when they rode over the burial mound,
they were resolute when they rode over the land.
Shield yourself now, you can escape this attack!
Out, little spear, if you are herein!
(I) stood under a lime-wood (shield), under a bright shield,
where the mighty women consulted their power,
and they sent screaming spears.
I will send another back to them,
a flying dart from the front in return.
Out, little spear, if it be herein! ...
If there be herein a piece of iron,
the work of witches, it must melt.
If you were shot in the skin, or were shot in the flesh,
or were shot in the blood,
or were shot in the limb, never may your life be harmed.
If it were gods' shot, or it were elves' shot,
or it were witches' shot, now I will help you.
This to you as a cure for gods' shot, this to you as a cure for elves' shot,
this to you as a cure for witches' shot; I will help you.
It is fleeing there on the mountaintop.
Be whole! May the Lord help you.)

Illness is a battlefield conflict, in which the patient has suffered a defeat by weapon-bearing, feminine supernatural warriors. The 'spear' causing the patient's pain represents an obvious penetration of the flesh, undone when the physician engages the 'mighty women' in combat and eventually banishes the spear back to the wilderness space from which its original wielders emerged. Falling sick is an act of unwilling submission to a superior opponent – but, by the same token, the resulting battle takes place on as grand a scale as a fight against literal invaders, reestablishing and policing the boundaries of the patient's body with the intensity of a military rout. Similarly, outside the medical corpus, illness is depicted as the placing of metaphorical bonds, fetters, or weights on a person, suggesting that disease – like sorrow, old age, extreme cold, and poverty – was understood to involve or evoke oppression and restriction, and to have recognisable commonalities with a state of captivity, servitude, and loss of personal bodily autonomy.[126] One medical

---

[125] *Lacnunga* no. 127.

[126] For example, *Andreas* ll. 577–81; *Guthlac B* ll. 881–8; *Christ III* ll. 1349–58. See Cavell, *Weaving Words*, 195–218.

charm in *Lacnunga* refers to a monstrous creature placing literal bonds, traces, or harnesses on a victim.[127]

Another medical charm that sends a disease agent back to the wilderness and away from human bodies and spaces uses a different metaphor to indicate invasion, violation, and breaching. The remedy is for a wen, like the salve discussed earlier. Here, too, a wen is a disease that has literally gotten under one's skin, a visible mark of the presence of something unwanted in the body. A wen under the skin and a wen on the heart differ only in the degree to which the swollen disease agent has penetrated into the body; it is a question not of what kind of malicious force seeks to enter the flesh, but how far it has progressed. The charm presents the sentient disease agent as a parasite:

> Wenne, wenne, wenchichenne,
> her ne scealt þu timbrien, ne nenne tun habben
> ac þu scealt north eonene to þan nihgan berhge
> þer þu hauest, ermig, enne broþer. . . .
> Clinge þu alswa col on heorþe
> scring þu alswa scerne awage
> and weorne alswa weter on anbre.[128]

> Wen, wen, wen-chicken,
> here you must not build, nor have a dwelling,
> but you must go from hence north to the nearby hill,
> there you have, miserable wretch, one brother. . . .
> May you shrink up, just like coal on the hearth,
> may you dry up, just like dung on a wall,
> and fade away, just like water in a vessel.

The *wenn* seeks to construct a *tun* (homestead, enclosed dwelling) inside the patient's body – what should be the patient's own most personal, private, and intimate 'enclosed dwelling'. The metaphor here is one of colonisation and settlement. The *wenn* builds a mockery of early medieval English home life, a kind of malicious parody or inversion of human community, and creates its own enclosure within an already-enclosed space from which it should rightly be expelled. Indeed, imagery associated with the early medieval English *tun* – pails of water, coals on the hearth, chickens – is used to shrink and belittle the *wenn*, which is banished not only from its own inappropriate homestead but also from all social and domestic spaces. Like the spear in *Wið færstice*, it must be sent back to a mountain or hill where its proper kin lives. As the boundaries of the patient's body are restored, the lines between human and non-human, *tun* and wilderness, are redrawn. Scholars have noted the tendency in Old English literature to treat the

---

[127] *Lacnunga* no. 86.
[128] London, British Library, Royal MS 4 A xiv f. 106v; the edition is *Metrical Charm 12* ll. 1–4, 8–10.

natural world as fundamentally hostile to humanity, a consequence of the disruption of the harmonious relationship between man and creation generated by the Fall.[129] These disease agents – spear-wielding women, the 'loathsome one that travels throughout the land', the *wenn* and its sibling – are not merely individual or personal threats, but representatives of all dangerous forces opposed to humanity and to the Christian God in a postlapsarian world.

The medical texts also fleetingly suggest that the violation of the body by disease could be metaphorically understood as an act of sexual violence. The medical corpus contains three mentions of a disease agent called a *mære*, who is described as 'riding' her victims. Old English glossaries consistently use the term *mære* to gloss the unusual Latin word *incuba*, a feminised form of the word *incubus*. The gloss is derived from Isidore's *Etymologiae*, which defines an *incubus* as a sexual demon who rapes its victims.[130] The presence of the *mære* in the *Leechbooks* and the treatment of her 'riding' as a sickness in and of itself draw an explicit conceptual equivalence between illness and sexual assault. Indeed, the medical texts hint at multiple types of erotic night demons: *Leechbook III* contains instructions for a salve operating 'wið ælfcynne ⁊ nihtgengan ⁊ þam mannum þe deofol mid hæmð' (for elf-kind and night-walkers and those people the devil has intercourse with).[131] The devil's sexual predations apparently either cause illness or empower the people so afflicted to injure others. Remedies for the *mære* also address other incursive disease agents and forces, including elvish 'influence' (*ælfsiden*), the 'night-walkers' mentioned earlier (*nihtgengan*), and the temptations or afflictions of demons.[132] If certain diseases were understood to be caused by the aggressive incursion of a supernatural agent, the forced submission of the human victim could be understood as an act of physical violence, as in the martial metaphors already discussed, or an act of eroticised violence.

What all these images have in common – from battlefield defeat to colonisation of the flesh to forced intercourse – is that they treat disease as a zero-sum power exchange and a near-complete loss of human autonomy, threatening the integrity of the entire body. This model of sickness has striking implications, in turn, for the concept of health, and the ways a healthy body is expected to look and function.

Hal *and* Unhal: *Whole, Holy, Healthy*

If sickness was indeed treated by many Old English medical texts as an anomalous dysfunction on the part of an imagined body that otherwise existed in a 'normative' state of integrity and functionality, and if sickness could – at

---

[129] See, for example, Neville, *Representations*; Magennis, *Images*.
[130] See further Batten, 'Dark Riders'.   [131] *Leechbook III*, ch. 61; see also ch. 54.
[132] *Bald's Leechbook I*, ch. 64; *Leechbook III*, ch. 1.

least in some remedies – be understood as a result of violation by the malevolent supernatural, we should expect to see evidence that its opposite, health, was thought to be a state of invulnerable wholeness safeguarded by God. The crux of this concept is the Old English adjective *hal* and related noun *hælu*, the words used to refer to health in the medical texts. These terms appear more than a hundred and thirty times in the medical corpus,[133] suggesting the importance of the concepts they convey to early medieval English understandings of the body, the practice of medicine, and the treatment of illness. The primary meaning of *hal* in the Old English corpus is 'whole, undivided', or 'entire, lacking no part'. In some cases, the term specifically means 'undamaged' or 'free from physical defect', while in religious verse and prose it also means 'safe from spiritual danger' or 'under the protection of God'.[134] *Hælu*, similarly, means 'good health', 'safety', and 'spiritual deliverance or salvation'.[135] The medical texts use the word *hal* and its opposite *unhal* – not whole, not healthy, damaged – to make fundamental distinctions of kind, between healthy and unhealthy patients, between living and dead flesh.[136] This conflation of health with wholeness, the erasure of damage, and holiness also permeates other medical vocabulary: the word *bot* means 'cure', 'healing', or 'remedy' in the medical texts, but also refers to compensation paid for infractions of the law or received for injury; atonement or penance for sin; relief or deliverance from suffering both physical and spiritual; and the literal repair or restoration of material objects.[137]

To be healthy in early medieval England, then, was literally to be 'all in one piece'. Health is the maintenance of the self as a continuous, invulnerable whole, without injury, defect, or point of entry. Physical wholeness also entails safety from spiritual threats, a state of being infused with the salvific protection of Christ. God's protection consists precisely of the maintenance of wholeness in the face of invasion. Latin supplications called *loricae*, 'breastplate' prayers, appear several times in the Old English medical corpus and in religious texts that contain remedies in their margins or prefatory material.[138] The speaker requests that God guard the entirety of their body, listed part by part, including individual internal organs. The speaker preserves his health by inviting God to permeate his flesh, shielding the body from penetration by malicious forces. In particular, the *Lorica of Laidcenn*, a Hiberno-Latin prayer popular in early medieval England, asks God to guard each of the body parts of the speaker in

---

[133] *Dictionary of Old English Corpus*, Simple Search, Cameron Number B21, 'Hal', 'Hæl-'.

[134] *Dictionary of Old English A to I* s.v. 'Hal'.

[135] *Dictionary of Old English A to I* s.v. 'Hælu'.

[136] For example, *Leechbook I*, chs. 32, 35; *Leechbook II*, ch. 58.

[137] *Dictionary of Old English A to I* s.v. 'Bot'.   [138] See further Hill, 'Invocation'.

turn and to protect the flesh as a whole from invasion – being torn open by devils and pierced with Satan's arrows – with his divine *inpenetrabile tutela* (impenetrable protection), glossed in Old English as *unþurhsceotendlicre gescyldnesses* (defence that cannot be shot through).[139] Ritual remedies also call on other symbols of wholeness and inviolacy to protect the patient: the use of milk from *unmæle* (unmarked, single-colour) cows, the employment of virgins as ritual assistants, and references to the perfected, fleshless, 'resurrection bodies' given to the faithful when they rise from the grave at Judgment Day all attest to the importance of maintaining the inviolate self in order to maintain health.[140] Indeed, the Christian emphasis on virginity is emphatically about wholeness in the Old English vocabulary: virgins of all genders are *unmæle* and *ungewemmed* – unspotted, uncorrupted, uninjured – and *gesund*, sound and entire. When physical and spiritual suffering overlap, medicine can be seen as linked to Christian devotional practice, an act of warding the body against the enemies of God and mankind and an invocation of Christian fleshly transcendence.[141]

These themes are also apparent in the ways Old English literary texts approach the body. Poetic terms for the body describe it as a closed container, a defended and defensible residence: it is the *banhus* (bone-house), *bancofa* (bone-chamber), and *ferðloca* (life-enclosure) containing the *sawelhord* (soul-treasure). The consequences of breaching the container can be dire. A number of poems refer to death and injury as the breaking open of the bodily structure or shell, the breaching of boundaries to sever life from the flesh.[142] The idea of the body being laid open for consumption also consistently preoccupies Old English religious texts. In the grave, the body is chewed by greedy worms, as noted earlier; descriptions of uncorrupted saintly corpses escaping that fate, and the transmutation of rotting bones into transparent, radiant resurrection bodies offer contrasting images of the ideal wholeness ordinary flesh cannot achieve. Vivid depictions of man-eating and cannibalism also mark the monsters of pre-Conquest literature, from Beowulf's famous enemy Grendel to the hybrid creatures described in *Wonders of the East*. One of the most common poetic motifs in Old English verse is that of 'the beasts of battle', a formulaic description of birds and wolves eager to consume the slain on battlefields, turning human bodies into carrion. These texts are also concerned with projectile intrusion: the devil, for example, is often described as assaulting humanity with darts, arrows, and iron weapons that metaphorically penetrate the flesh

---

[139] *Lacnunga* no. 65, l. 27.

[140] See, for example, *Lacnunga* nos. 29, 63, 64, 86, 163, 176; *Herbarium*, ch. 104.2.

[141] Jolly, 'Margins', 136; Gay, 'Incantations', 34–5.

[142] Cavell, *Weaving Words*, 207–16. See, for example, *Andreas* ll. 1238, 1404; *Fortunes of Men* l. 33; *Guthlac B* ll. 954–63, 1027–33; *Beowulf* ll. 2422, 2501, 3143.

and injure the soul with sin.[143] The *Prose Dialogue of Solomon and Saturn*, one of three Christian esoteric texts recounting dialogues between the biblical King Solomon and the prince of the Chaldeans, describes devils penetrating the mouths, skin, flesh, and bowels of unwary men and using their bodies as a kind of lightning rod to travel into the earth towards Hell.[144] The profusion of these collected examples suggests a profound cultural preoccupation with bodily integrity and bodily wholeness.

Illuminating these early medieval English attitudes towards the body, however, begs an essential question: what does a model that conflates healthiness with wholeness – with the potentially troubling idea of being 'undamaged' – mean for people with physical or bodily differences and impairments? What did it mean to be 'abled' or 'disabled' in early medieval England, and what can the textual, historical, and archaeological records tell us about both the lives of disabled persons and the way that 'disability' was understood and discussed in literature, medicine, law, and religious thought? The following section seeks to address these questions and their complex, multifaceted answers.

Impairment and Disability

The Welsh monk Asser, in his biography of Alfred the Great, describes the king as the best of warriors, devoted to his education, courageous as a wild boar, a builder of cities, and a consummate diplomat – and the sufferer of numerous illnesses unknown to physicians. Alfred, Asser tells us, had prayed to God to grant him an infirmity 'quam posset sustinere' (that he could tolerate) to help restrain his carnal desires, but which would not render him 'indignum et inutilem in mundanis rebus' (unworthy and useless in worldly affairs).[145] He is soon afflicted by *ficus*, a disease that is difficult for modern scholars to identify but which may have been haemorrhoids.[146] Plagued by this ailment, Alfred asks for divine mercy:

> ... diu in oratione tacita prostratus, ita Domini misericordiam
> deprecabatur, quatenus omnipotens Deus pro sua immense
> clementia stimulos praesentis et infestantis infirmitatis aliqua
> qualicunque leviori infirmitate mutaret, ea tamen condicione,
> ut corporaliter exterius illa infirmitas non appareret, ne inutilis
> et despectus esset. Timebat enim lepram aut caccitatem, vel
> aliquem talem dolorem, qui homines tam cito et inutiles et
> despectos suo adventu efficiunt.

---

[143] *Beowulf* ll. 1741–4; *Guthlac B* ll. 1141–5; *Juliana* ll. 468–72; *Christ II* ll. 766–9; *Vainglory* l. 27; Bede, *Historia Ecclesiastica*, V.13. See Atherton, 'Figure of the Archer'.
[144] *Prose Dialogue of Solomon and Saturn*, ll. 42–49.   [145] Asser, *Life of King Alfred*, ch. 74.
[146] Kershaw, 'Illness', 209.

> ... he lay in silent prayer a long while, in order to beseech the
> Lord's mercy, that Almighty God in his bountiful kindness
> might substitute for the pangs of the present and agonising
> infirmity some less severe illness, on the understanding that
> the new illness would not be outwardly visible on his body,
> whereby he would be rendered useless and contemptible. For
> he feared leprosy or blindness, or some other such disease,
> which so quickly render men useless and contemptible by their
> onslaught.[147]

Alfred is consequently struck by severe internal pain at his wedding feast, which replaces his *ficus* but assails him for the rest of his life. Alfred's suffering, and his constant fear that the pain would return, 'quasi inutilem eum, ut ei videtur, in divinis et humanis rebus propemodum effecit' (rendered him as if virtually useless, as it seemed to him, in heavenly and worldly affairs), but he continues to prove himself on the battlefield and as a ruler. His tribulations, according to Asser, only make his political success more impressive and demonstrate his martyr-like capacity for endurance and faith.

This narrative provides a rich case study for discussions of impairment and disability in early medieval England. Alfred's greatest concerns are that he will have a *visible* disease – that is, an illness that disrupts the integrity of his body as a unified whole – and that his condition, like (apparently) blindness and leprosy in other people, will render him useless and unworthy of respect. Asser's constant, laboured repetition that Alfred seeks specifically to avoid becoming *inutilis* and that he is only useless in his own perception (*quasi ... ut ei videtur ... propemodum*) suggests that a contemporary audience would otherwise have been inclined to see Alfred's chronically ill body as a sign of unfitness, unworthiness, or contemptibility.[148] The worst thing a king can be, apparently, is ineffective. Asser's repeated emphasis on Alfred's battlefield prowess and courage compensates narratively for his illness. Yet Alfred's body is also a tool of political power. His ability to persevere through an ailment that threatens to limit his power and diminish his social status – that would, in other words, be disabling – demonstrates his Christian devotion and his superhuman leadership. His illness is a mode of self-discipline, a way of modelling Christian and secular virtue, service, and sacrifice. Alfred's bodily pain must be kept invisible to maintain his worthiness but revealed at certain moments to allow praise of his strength and self-control; he is sick enough to be righteous, but well enough to maintain his position of social dominance.[149] Alfred the Great is, to use a term coined by disability activists, a 'supercrip': a man treated

---

[147] Asser, *Life of King Alfred*, ch. 74; translation from Keynes and Lapidge, *Alfred the Great*, 89.
[148] Kershaw, 'Illness', 210; Pratt, 'Illnesses', 56.   [149] Crawford, 'Differentiation', 96.

as worthy of admiration because he succeeds in spite of his impairments, which are assumed to be oppressive burdens antithetical to his thriving.

These themes resonate throughout the Old English and Anglo-Latin textual corpus in depictions and discussions of impaired people. Impairment is treated as a burden, a source of oppression, a manifestation of original sin, a trial sent by God to purify his chosen favourites, and an opportunity for the non-impaired to demonstrate charity and for saints to perform miracles. Always, however, impairment is treated as the absence of, or an obstacle to, individual and social power or agency.

Concepts of Impairment and Ability in Early Medieval England

The field of disability studies has long operated on a set of assumptions known as the 'social model' of disability: *impairment* describes an organic physical or mental condition[150] that inhibits or alters bodily function, while *disability* is socially constructed – the barriers, disadvantages, and instances of exclusion an individual with an impairment encounters.[151] The cultural model of disability revises and builds upon this social model to assert that disability is 'largely but not strictly synonymous with sites of cultural oppression', an interaction between social obstacles and biological capacities.[152] Impairment is as culturally constructed as disability: physical difference is not ontological or 'purely' natural, but created through encounters in which a person has meaning imposed upon their body.[153] Ability, too, is culturally determined and context-dependent. There is no singular societal response to impairment and no singular definition of ability; both must be observed within their cultural context and without *a priori* assumptions about their nature.

In Old English, however, there is no word for 'disability' as an identity, community, or broad category of experience, and very little evidence of any kind of disabled culture.[154] The mutability of impairment as a cultural signifier essentially defies the imposition of any single model. The present discussion distinguishes between impairment and disability because it can be difficult to determine which impairments would have had disabling consequences for early medieval English individuals, and what those consequences would have been. Certain kinds of impairment were likely more common in pre-Conquest England than in present-day Western Europe, and thus some conditions we

---

[150] I use the word 'condition' in this section of necessity, to mean 'circumstance' or 'state of being'. There are very few ways of speaking about impairment and disability currently available to us that have not developed pathologising connotations, which I do not intend to convey and actively disavow.

[151] Shakespeare, 'Social Model'.   [152] Snyder and Mitchell, *Cultural Locations*, 7–10.

[153] See Brownlee, 'Perceptions', 54.   [154] Singer, 'Disability', 135–7.

might now consider 'bodily difference' may have been considered part of the course of ordinary life. A great deal of socially essential labour is available to, or can be adjusted for, persons with impairments, so certain impairments might have been disabling in some ways but not in others.[155]

Old English terms for individual impairments survive – for example, one may be *blind*, *deaf*, *dumb*, or assigned a catch-all term for those with mobility impairments, words whose modern descendants have come to be used as profound insults (*lam*, 'lame'; *healte*, 'halt'; *crypol*, 'cripple', 'one who crawls'). One might fall somewhere on a spectrum of 'ill hearing' or have 'dim' and 'misty' eyes.[156] Blindness, deafness, and mobility impairments are often grouped together in Old English prose and verse as conditions that mark the suffering of humanity on earth and that can be healed by Christ and his saints – but such groupings follow biblical convention, rather than necessarily testifying to an understanding of these impairments as belonging to a single, recognised social category.[157] Instead the sources contain words that refer to illness, impairment, and injury as contiguous and overlapping states, without differentiating between acute and chronic. The most common terms used are *unhal* and *unhælu*, discussed in the previous section. Illness and impairment are both a state of un-wholeness, of damage and vulnerability. Depictions of the long-term sick and impaired, which are found most commonly in saints' lives describing healing miracles, often emphasise the 'leakiness' of these bodies: they swell up, emit effluvia, have open wounds, and manifest ulcers and tumours. Their ailments disrupt their visual and conceptual wholeness. The medical texts use the word *unhal* to refer to anyone who is currently sick and seeking medical attention; lawcodes and hagiography use the term to refer to anyone who deviates, for a short or long period of time, from a standard of bodily strength, functionality, and completeness that is positioned as normative.[158] Another word used in this way is *untrumnesse* (lit. 'un-firmness'), while multiple lawcodes use *unmiht* (lit. 'un-strength', 'un-power') and *unmaga* (lit. 'un-strong', unable) to refer to persons who are legally dependent on others, including the old, the very young, the poor, and those with a range of physical impairments.[159] The repeated use of negating prefixes in these terms suggests that sickness and impairment were understood to be an *absence* of health, strength, power, and

---

[155] Lee, 'Abled', 41–3.

[156] See, for example, the various remedies in *Bald's Leechbook I*, chs. 2–3; on the spectrum of hearing loss, see Garner, 'Deaf Studies'.

[157] For example, Ælfric, 'Of the Catholic Faith' (ed. Clemoes, *Homilies*), ll. 248–9, 'Third Sunday after Pentecost' (ed. Godden, *Homilies*), ll. 77–81; *Life of St. Margaret* (ed. Clayton and Magennis), ch. 19; Vercelli Homily IV, ll. 194–202; *Andreas* ll. 577–84; *Elene* ll. 1213–15; *Solomon and Saturn I* ll. 77–9.

[158] Skevington, 'Unhal'.

[159] See *Dictionary of Old English Corpus*, Simple Search, 'Untrum-', 'Unmiht', 'Unmaga'.

wholeness – again positioning such health and strength as normative, with impairment treated as a deviation or defect. Some texts make this attitude explicit. The Old English *Boethius*, for example, describes walking as 'eallum monnum gecynde' (natural for all people), while those who cannot walk lack power over their bodies (*næfð his fota geweald*) – and everyone knows (*wat ælc man*) that a person who walks is stronger (*mihtigra*) than one who crawls. The walking man, the text reveals, is a metaphor for a good person who desires, and moves, *on riht* (rightly) and the crawling man is an evil person who desires, and moves, *on woh* (in error).[160] These moralising judgements about natural, correct bodies and unnatural, incorrect ones speak for themselves. Full humanity belongs to bodies that are 'whole'.

A number of late Old English lawcodes codify these oppositions between healthy and unhealthy, powerful and weak, and associate impairment with old age, dependent childhood, poverty, and slavery as conditions that include certain legal debilitations and also require certain degrees of legal protection.[161] VI Æthelred (c.1008) declares:

> Se maga and se unmaga ne beoð na gelice, ne ne magon na
> gelice byrþene ahebban, ne se unhala þe ma þam halum
> gelice; and þy man sceal medmian and gescadlice toscadan,
> ge on godcundan scriftan ge on woroldcundan steoran ylde
> and geogoþe, welan and wædle, hæle and unhæle, and hada
> gehwilcne ... se þe nydwyrhta bið þæs þe he misdeð se bið
> gebeorhges and þy beteran domes symle wyrðe þe he
> nydwyrhta wæs þæs þe he worhte.[162]

> The able and the unable are not alike, nor can they bear a
> like burden, any more than the unhealthy are like the healthy;
> and so one must take the measure and separately distinguish
> in both spiritual penance and in worldly punishment old age
> and youth, wealth and poverty, health and sickness, and each
> social rank ... the one who acts from necessity and so commits
> a misdeed is worthy of protection and easier judgments
> because he acted from compulsion.

The text goes on to group women, children, enslaved persons, and impaired persons in this way. II Cnut (c.1018) contains nearly the same proclamation, stressing that 'a man sceal unstrangam menn for godes lufe and ege liþelicor deman and scrifon þonne þam strangan' (one must, for love and fear of God, judge and penalise weak persons more gently than the strong).[163] Such articulations of complete and fundamental opposition between healthy and sick, strong and weak – without

---

[160] *Old English Boethius* 36.107–119.   [161] Rabin, 'Litigation', 278–9.
[162] VI Æthelred 52–52.1.   [163] II Cnut 68.

acknowledgement that an individual could move between states – are both protect-ive and restrictive, relegating entire classes of people to a form of legal dependency. The lawcodes make provision for impaired individuals, but also qualify their legal personhood, simultaneously including them in and excluding them from social and legal communities. *Unhal* serves as a broad category for bodies perceived as less capable, less powerful, entangled with other social markers of (dis)empowerment like gender and rank.

Despite the fact that illness and impairment are treated as an absence of health, the *hal* body – whole, holy, healthy – is almost always defined in comparison to and in the context of bodies that lack *hælu*, the presence of health only made visible by its absence. In the medical texts, health is simply the amelioration or eradication of sickness; a patient 'bið sona hal' (will soon be whole) if the remedy is effectively deployed. The lawcodes of Æthelberht and Alfred offer long lists of the varying amounts of monetary compensation owed to a person if damage is done to each of their body parts.[164] Æthelberht assigns fifty shillings – the same price demanded for the killing of a free man – to the loss of eyes and of hearing, injuries to the shoulders, the loss of a foot, and destruction of the genitals. Alfred's lawcode concurs that castration, the loss of the leg or foot, and wounds to the eyes and shoulders command the greatest compensation, along with damage to the hands and to the sinews of the leg and neck. The fact that these injuries merit financial compensation suggests both that the default body is expected to have two eyes that can see, two ears that can hear, shoulders that can lift and rotate, two legs that enable walking, two hands with ten fingers that can grip items, and so forth, with the loss or alteration of these body parts representing a grave detri-ment, and also that such loss or alteration might have economic consequences for the individual against which reparative payment is a bulwark. The normative body comes into view at the moment it is rendered non-normative.

This 'itemised' body is also a marker of health and normativity in early medieval English religious literature and prayer. The *Lorica of Laidcenn*, the protective prayer discussed in the previous section, asks God to preserve more than a hundred of the speaker's discrete body parts, including at least thirty-three individual parts of the head and face (nose, nostrils, pupils, irises, gums, teeth, epiglottis, etc.).[165] A similar Latin prayer in *Lacnunga* banishes the devil from eleven individual body parts and from 'ab uniuersis confaginibus membrorum eis' (the whole framework of [the patient's] members).[166] An exhaustive excom-munication formula similarly expels a person from the Christian community by

---

[164] Æthelberht 33–73; Alfred 44–77. See further Richards, 'Body', and Oliver, *Body Legal*, chs. 2–6.
[165] *Lacnunga* no. 65.
[166] *Lacnunga* no. 63. See also *Leechbook III*, ch. 62, the Leofric Missal (ed. Orchard, 438), and the margins of Corpus Christi College MS 41, p. 292.

cursing each of their body parts in turn, including eyes, ears, tongue, lips, windpipe, shoulders, chest, feet, and legs, while a confessional formula instructs the penitent to confess all the sins committed by their eyes, ears, mouth, skin, flesh, bone, sinew, vein, gristle, hair, and marrow.[167] Ælfric of Eynsham, in a homily for the fourth Sunday after Easter, explains that Christ's followers knew he had been truly resurrected in body because they could witness all of his functioning parts:

> Ealle his lima he hæfde, and hæfð butan twyn; on his fotum he stod, and þa næron butan sceancan; his sidan hy grapodon, and he soðlice hæfde ge innoð ge breost, butan þam þe ne magon ænige sidan beon to geswuteligenne. Innoð he hæfde eac, þa ða he æt and dranc; and tungan he hæfde, þa ða he to him spræc; and he næs butan toðum, þe mid þære tungan swegdon; and þrotan he hæfde, þa ða hy gehyrdon his stæmne; and his handa hæfdon, þe hy gegrapedon, earmas and exla, on ansundum lichaman.[168]

> He had all his limbs, and has without doubt; on his feet he stood, and they were not without the lower leg; his sides they examined, and he truly had both internal organs and a breast, except for those which cannot have any surface to show. Internal organs he had also, when he ate and drank; and he had a tongue, when he spoke to them; and he was not without teeth, which made sound with the tongue; and he had a throat, when they heard his voice; and his hands – which they gripped – had arms and shoulders, on a sound body.

Christ's body is *ansund* (sound, whole, entire) because it has the correct number of components and because all of those components function as they should and operate collaboratively: teeth, tongue, and throat; hands, arms, and shoulders; inside and outside. Indeed, Ælfric's insistence that Christ's digestive system and larynx were operating correctly after his resurrection draws attention to a perpetual theme in early medieval English discussions of health, sickness, and impairment: the importance of function, and what Asser calls *utilitas*. Æthelberht and Alfred's lawcodes increase compensation for injuries that impair function: hearing, sight, walking, gripping, rotating the shoulders, and holding up one's own head and neck.[169] Æthelberht's lawcode states that full compensation – the same as for a death – should be paid if a servant loses an eye or a foot, presumably because such a loss would diminish their capacity to serve.[170] Saints' lives describe numerous impaired people seeking healing from relics and at shrines, and the emphasis is always on what these people cannot do – see, hear, speak, walk, sit up, move their limbs.

---

[167] Texts in Treharne, 'Excommunication'; Fowler, 'Handbook', 17–18.
[168] Ælfric, 'Fourth Sunday after Easter' (ed. Pope, *Supplement*), ll. 145–61.
[169] Richards, 'Body', 112.   [170] Æthelberht 87.

The normative, healthy body is thus a unity assembled from a long list of individual parts that all must operate correctly and collaboratively, with particular importance attached to eyes, ears, speech organs, shoulders, hands, the abdomen with innards, and legs with feet.[171] Any one of those parts failing to operate at full capacity within the whole – or indeed ceasing to be – is a detriment to the integrity of the body and constitutes both an impairment and, potentially, a disability. Indeed, the Old English *Boethius* notes that if the body is missing a limb, 'þonne be bið hit no full mon swa hit ær wæs' (then it is no longer as complete a person as it once was).[172] The healthy body is not just an assemblage, of course: its visual and conceptual wholeness remains important. Visible wounds and scars explicitly merit higher compensation in the lawcodes than ones that can be hidden.[173] Alfred was apparently desperate not to have an illness outwardly visible on his flesh. Even Christ's side wound, which his followers behold as proof that he died, is described in Ælfric's homily for the fourth Sunday after Easter as only a *dolhswæþ* (scar, trace; l. 142): the holy, resurrected body is marked but has no vulnerable gape. The body must be closed and complete, as discussed in the previous section – but this completeness also depends on all individual members being present and accounted for. In Exeter Book Riddle 82, the solution to which is 'a one-eyed garlic seller', the person's single eye does as much work to signify non-normativity as their *twelf hund heafda* (twelve hundred heads): too many heads, the riddle indicates, and too few eyes, with the phrases *an eage* and *twelf hund heafda* framing a list of 'normal' numbers of ears, feet, hands, arms, and shoulders.

This evident bias against impaired bodies in the textual record, however, does not suggest banishment, ostracism, or total exclusion of impaired persons from social communities. Impairment was evidently considered an undesirable state, but the lawcodes make provision for *unhal* people within social and legal structures, not outside of them. An emphasis on function provides opportunities for the economic and social contributions that impaired persons can make to their communities to be considered 'normative'.[174] A number of studies on the 'history of disability' assume that the Middle Ages was a period of unrelenting persecution for persons with impairments,[175] but the archaeological and textual records suggest instead complex and varied attitudes towards people with bodily differences and a range of experiences for those people within their communities.

---

[171] See also Sweany, 'Imagination', 99–105.   [172] *Old English Boethius* 37.86–7 (see also 34).
[173] O'Brien O'Keeffe, 'Body and Law', 215; Oliver, *Body Legal*, 165–79; see, for example, Alfred 45.1, 49, 66.1.
[174] Brownlee, 'Perceptions', 54.   [175] Metzler, *Disability*, 13–18.

Disabled Persons in the Historical Record

Early medieval English cemeteries from the sixth to the eleventh centuries include individuals with a variety of conditions that might have caused them impairment in life. The burial record attests to persons with osteoarthritis of differing degrees, tuberculosis, leprosy, limb differences of many kinds including fractures and other trauma, paralysis, cleft palate, spinal morphologies that could affect posture, movement, and body shape, various types of neuromuscular differences, hydrocephaly, cancers, Paget's disease, deafness, and numerous other bodily conditions, including signs of osteomyelitis and inflammation that may be the result of any number of illnesses.[176] Graves have also survived of individuals with dwarfism, gigantism, and facial differences. This list is not complete. Experiences of pain or loss of function can be hard to determine from skeletal remains alone, and the list necessarily does not include conditions of the soft tissue, like blindness, that undoubtedly existed in the population. In addition, very little can be gleaned about intellectual disabilities in early medieval England from either the textual or archaeological record. Words that may reflect the existence of intellectual disabilities, like *ungewit* or *dysgunge*, are elided with terms for mental illness.[177] The *Life of St Margaret* describes Margaret's blessing on households as preventing the birth of 'nan unhal cild . . . ne crypol, ne dumb, ne deaf, ne blind, ne ungewittes' (no unhealthy child . . . neither mobility-impaired, nor mute, nor deaf, nor blind, nor without wits), the last item of which seems to refer to intellectual disability, but otherwise the evidence is thin.[178] Madness itself (*wod*), which probably refers to multiple conditions, is treated as disabling in hagiography and occasionally also included in lists of impairments.[179]

In addition, conditions and experiences that we would not consider impairments may have been treated as such: menstruation is described as a form of *untrumness*, as is pregnancy, suggesting a distrust of such bodies bound up in early medieval English understandings of sex and gender.[180] Old age, too, is described as socially disabling – to become old, according to homilies and religious verse, is by definition to acquire numerous impairments – and death is treated as the ultimate impairment of the body, blinding the eyes, deafening the ears, and paralysing the feet and hands.[181] The continuum of ability on which real, embodied people in early medieval England lived defies the clean separations between *hal* and *unhal* that the Old English lawcodes and medical texts seek to enforce.

---

[176] Brownlee, 'Perceptions', 59; Bohling, 'Death', 87.

[177] For example, *Bald's Leechbook I*, ch. 66.   [178] *Life of St Margaret*, ch. 19.

[179] For example, Ælfric, 'Of the Catholic Faith', l. 249.

[180] Bruce Wallace, 'Intersections'; see Bede, *Historia ecclesiastica*, I.27.

[181] For example, Vercelli Homily IX, ll. 79–82, 89–98; *Soul and Body*. See Porck, *Old Age*, 76–109; Parker, 'Embodied Lives', 19.

Accessing the experience of persons with impairments in early medieval England is difficult, but we can draw a handful of reasonable conclusions from the available evidence. The majority of burials of impaired persons are in central locations within cemeteries and have been given normative rites, including features of burial that seem to prioritise the comfort of the corpse, like carefully propping up paralysed limbs.[182] Such a lack of differentiation means that these people were integrated into their communities – or at least that they were not so discriminated against in life that they faced exclusion in death. It is important to note, however, that a disproportionately high number of non-normative burials are of impaired persons, particularly notable in a period in which burial is generally standardised, and by some counts around 30–40 per cent of excavated graves of impaired individuals are non-normative burials or are found in marginal locations.[183] Some early cemeteries have noticeable spatial associations between impaired persons, non-adults, and skeletons that archaeologists have sexed female; these patterns lessen in the later pre-Conquest period.[184] Distinctive burials are hard to interpret, but generally suggest some kind of differentiation in life.

Many graves of impaired persons show signs that they lived with and managed their illness or impairment: adults with conditions that would have been present since childhood, evidence of healed amputations and fractures, impaired persons who lived into old age. Survival does not necessarily indicate compassion or acceptance, but in some cases these individuals lived with impairments that would have required care, which they evidently received.[185] Saints' lives often describe impaired persons visiting shrines with the assistance of kin and friends. Alfred's lawcode contains a telling provision: 'Gif hwa oðrum his unmagan oðfæste, and he hine on ðære fæstinge forferie, getriowe hine facnes se ðe hine fede, gif hine hwa hwelces teo' (If someone entrusts his dependant/unable person to another, and he [the dependant] dies during that time of fostering, he who sustained him is to clear himself of guilt, if anyone accuses him of any crime).[186] This suggests that some impaired people received care in their communities, that such care was expected to ensure the survival of those people, and that sometimes their care was insufficient. Accounts of wealthy impaired persons with access to resources describe them as relying on servants to move about. Saints' lives also describe individuals being carried on litters or by friends, as well as using crutches, staves, and stools, and blind

---

[182] Brownlee, 'Perceptions', 56–7; Hadley, 'Burying', 110–11; Bohling, 'Death'; Lee, 'Disease', 713.
[183] Brownlee, 'Perceptions', 62; Hadley, 'Burying', 104–5; Bohling, 'Death', 599.
[184] Bohling, 'Death', 345.   [185] Brownlee, 'Perceptions', 57; Bohling, 'Death', 555.
[186] Alfred 17.

persons are described as having or hiring guides.[187] The Anglo-French monk Lantfred included in his *Translation and Miracles of Saint Swithun* accounts of people with impairments helping one another on their journeys to Swithun's shrine in Winchester (e.g. a man who could not speak serving as a guide for three blind women), suggesting perhaps a nascent concept of community among people with physical impairments.[188] Other individuals undoubtedly managed without care from others, whether by choice or necessity.

Some impairments probably had relatively little impact on a person's social position and economic role, even if they affected daily life. The high-status Castledyke burial of a woman who would have been at least partially deaf in life suggests that she was a wife and mother, for example, and would likely have been able to engage in important economic and cultural labour like weaving.[189] Other impairments would have impacted a person's ability to participate fully as an adult member of society. Some lawcodes impose fines on free men for neglecting military service. Cnut's lawcode is adamant that to be a legal witness, a man must be able to see and hear. Alfred's lawcode declares that 'Gif mon sie dumb oððe deaf geboren, þæt he ne mæge synna onsecgan ne geandettan, bete se fæder his misdæda' (If a person is born mute or deaf, so that he may neither deny nor confess his sins, let his father make reparations for his misdeeds).[190] Paired with the declarations that the *hal* and *unhal* cannot be treated alike under the law, these provisions collectively suggest that an adult man who could not walk and ride a horse, carry weapons, see, hear, or speak might well be prohibited from participating in essential aspects of social and political life.[191] Certain impairments may also have prevented one from holding public office, especially royal and war leadership, as Asser and Alfred's shared anxiety suggests; attempts to blind rival heirs to the throne indicate that impairment might have lessened one's eligibility to rule.[192] In the entry for 1055, the *Anglo-Saxon Chronicle* also notes that Bishop Æthelstan was replaced because he was *unfere* (infirm, feeble, incapacitated), a word that elsewhere refers to a lack of health, strength, and social power.[193]

---

[187] Bede, *Historia Ecclesiastica*, IV.8, IV.10; Lantfred, *Translatio et Miracula* (ed. Lapidge, *Cult*), ch. 18; *Anonymous Life of Cuthbert* (ed. Colgrave, *Two Lives*), IV.5; for numerous other examples in *vitae*, see Lee, 'Disability', 30.

[188] For example, Lantfred, *Translatio et Miracula*, ch. 5.

[189] Bruce Wallace, 'Intersections', 46; Hadley, 'Burying', 111.

[190] Ine 51; II Cnut 23; Alfred 14. Alfred's description of deaf and mute people as being unable to deny or confess sins raises the possibility that both conditions were thought to overlap with intellectual disability. See Metzler, *Fools*, 54.

[191] Crawford, 'Differentiation', 95.

[192] *Chronicle MS C* (ed. O'Brien O'Keeffe), 1036; William of Malmesbury, *Gesta Regum Anglorum*, (ed. Mynors, Thomson, and Winterbottom), II.136–7. See O'Brien O'Keeffe, 'Body and Law', 212–14.

[193] *Chronicle MS C*, 1055.

For the ordinary person, however, the available evidence suggests that the degree to which an impairment could be socially disabling varied depending on economic status. High-status burials of impaired individuals suggest that impairment need not be an impediment to social status if one belonged to a wealthy and well-resourced kin network.[194] The relatively high number of impaired persons buried in non-normative graves, however, along with evident political and legal restrictions based on physical difference, frequent depictions of impaired persons as living in poverty in hagiography, and the textual treatment of impairment as an undesirable state suggest that if one was not well-resourced, impairment might have been one of several factors that could render one socially vulnerable and more likely to experience exclusion.[195] Two episodes in Bede provide an excellent example: Tortgyth, a noble-born nun, holds a position of significant power at Barking Abbey that she retains while experiencing paralysis and muteness, while a poor youth treated by John of Beverley for muteness and skin disease is destitute, abandoned by his community due to his impairment.[196] The degree to which impairments would have been disabling probably varied greatly between individuals depending both on the nature of the impairment and on social circumstance.

Literary Approaches to Sickness and Disability

Approaches to illness and impairment in medieval literature are 'manifold and ambiguous',[197] but distinct themes are traceable in the Old English corpus, most notably that impairment is consistently positioned as an absence of power. As we have already seen, impairment in the lawcodes, medical texts, and other literature is often treated as a detriment to the body that must be compensated for. Like sickness, it is also often described in Old English verse and prose as a form of bondage and torment, or a physical burden that oppresses the individual with its weight.[198] Other sources treat it as a tragic misfortune to be avoided: the person 'on feðe lef, / seonobennum seoc' (injured with respect to motion, sick with a sinew-wound) must 'sar cwanian, / murnan meotodges-ceaft' (lament his wound, mourn his meted-out condition).[199] The birth of children who are impaired in various ways – blind, deaf, unable to speak or walk – is cited as a punishment in several homilies for having intercourse on

---

[194] Lee, 'Abled', 44; Bruce Wallace, 'Intersections', 44–6; Bohling, 'Death', 238.

[195] Crawford, 'Differentiation', 94; Hadley, 'Burying', 111.

[196] Bede, *Historia ecclesiastica*, IV.9, V.2.   [197] Metzler, *Disability*, 47.

[198] For example, see Cavell, *Weaving Words*, 196–220. See also Ælfric, *Life of Swithun* (ed. Skeat, *Lives of Saints*), ll. 95–134.

[199] *Fortunes of Men* ll. 17–20. See also Ælfric, 'First Friday of Lent' (ed. Pope, *Supplement*), ll. 56–7.

Holy Sunday and fast days.[200] Prognostics offer strict dietary advice for expectant mothers so that their children are not born *disig* (stupid), *hoforode* (humpbacked), or *healede* (hydrocephalous), and one of the obstetric charms preserved in *Lacnunga* instructs the woman to banish the possibility of 'þære laðan lambyrde' (the loathsome 'lame' birth).[201] Though the Old English medical texts rarely blame illness on a person's individual actions – this language of maternal responsibility for neonatal health is perhaps an exception, though it also grants bodily control to expectant mothers even while implicitly attributing fault should this medical advice not be followed – religious texts do occasionally mention that disease and impairment can be evidence of or punishments for sin.[202] There is, however, relatively little emphasis on the idea of sickness as punishment across the corpus as a whole.[203] Far more often, impairments are used as metaphors for sin as a concept, as we have already seen in the *Boethius*. Didactic texts equate physical 'deficiencies' with spiritual ones: blindness as a metaphor for the inability to perceive religious truth, deafness as a metaphor for the refusal to listen to God's commands, and so forth.[204] Impairment here is not a symbol of individual sin, but of original sin. It becomes a shorthand for the ways in which humanity is estranged from God in a postlapsarian world, a sign of divine absence.[205] Illness and unhealthiness, early medieval English discussions of Genesis note, came into existence with the Fall; numerous homilies teach their audiences that God afflicts the bodies of mortal men because humanity has fallen from grace.[206] The impaired body is legible, available for use as a parable, a metonymic stand-in for all human suffering and imperfection.

Ælfric offers several possible aetiologies of impairment: 'hwilon for heora synnum, hwilon for fandunge; hwilon for godes wundrum, hwilon for geheald-sumnysse goddra drohtnunga; þæt hi þy eadmodran beon' (sometimes for their

---

[200]   Texts in Rudolf, 'Preaching', 52.

[201]   Tiberius A.iii Prognostic (ed. Chardonnens), ll. 20–22; *Lacnunga* no. 161. See Metzler, *Disability*, 85–9.

[202]   For example, see DiNapoli, *Index*, s.v. 'Blindness', 'Deafness', 'Disease', 'Lameness'; Bede, *Historia ecclesiastica* I.7, IV.21; Vercelli Homily XXII; Wulfstan, *Sermo Lupi ad Anglos* (ed. Bethurum, *Homilies*, 269).

[203]   Lee, 'Abled', 48; Thompson, *Dying*, 92.

[204]   See numerous homilies under DiNapoli's headwords in fn. 202, including Ælfric on the Feast Day of the Holy Martyrs, the first Friday in Lent, and the third Sunday after Pentecost; *Juliana* ll. 468–75; *Old English Soliloquies* (ed. Carnicelli), bk. 1; Bede, 'On Tobias' (ed. Foley and Holder, *Miscellany*).

[205]   On a similar theme in late medieval literature, see Wheatley, *Stumbling Blocks*. For discussion of this idea in the Old English corpus, see Parker, 'Embodied Lives'.

[206]   On the origin of illness and death, see *Genesis A* ll. 946–8; Bede, *In Genesim* (trans. Kendall, 128); *Guthlac B* ll. 850–72. On the imperfection of earthly bodies, see, for example, Vercelli Homily XXII; Ælfric, 'Passion of St Bartholomew', ll. 275–7. For discussion, Parker, 'Embodied Lives', 249, 299; Lee, 'Disability', 27–9.

sins, sometimes as a trial; sometimes for the miracles of God, sometimes for the preservation of good conduct; so that they might be more humble).[207] The same texts that use impairment as a metaphor for sin and human failure also treat the experience of impairment as a trial of faith, a mode of purifying the soul on earth, and a marker of special holiness given by God to test his favourites. The examples are numerous: St Cuthbert's endurance of an inflamed and foreshortened leg is proof of his self-discipline; the abbess Hild receives an illness from God 'so that her strength might be made perfect in infirmity' (*ut . . . uirtus eius in infirmitate perficeretur*); the abbess Æthelthryth endures a neck tumour to purge her soul of the sin of wearing necklaces in her youth; King Alfred, of course, is made a martyr and paragon of self-control by his illness, as is St Guthlac of Crowland, discussed in the next section.[208] Numerous homilies and religious texts, following the writings of various church fathers, explicitly state that sickness and impairment are a trial to be endured to obtain a place in heaven.[209] Impairment is thus used to signify membership in an exalted community of the pure and chosen, which undoubtedly confers a kind of social power – but that power is derived from the endurance of a condition that is only ever treated as a source of suffering, and from a willing submission to God and the embrace of a powerless state. Many of the figures experiencing holy impairment are treated by their texts as supercrips, worthy of admiration because they persevere through their illnesses and injuries.

The lawcodes, by contrast, treat the impaired body as a legible sign of both crime and criminality. The list of injuries meriting compensation means that the body is itself a witness to and evidence for the occurrence of a crime, but in many lawcodes mutilation is also a means of punishment and restitution. Hands and feet should be struck off, tongues cut out, eyes blinded, ears ripped from the head, and genitals removed as punishments for a variety of crimes including theft and rape.[210] The body becomes a site for the demonstration of the power of the king and his law, but the lawcodes also frame such punishment as an opportunity for the guilty person to purify their soul through the suffering of impairment, in much the same manner as the trials of holiness described earlier – here offered as torture, discipline, and gift by a secular authority in a supposed

---

[207] Ælfric, 'Passion of St Bartholomew', ll. 250–4.

[208] Bede, *Life of Cuthbert*, chs. II, VIII, XXIII, XXVIII, and *Historia ecclesiastica*, IV.19, IV.23.

[209] *Old English Pastoral Care* (ed. Sweet, 250); Ælfric, 'Feast Day of the Holy Martyrs', l. 292, 'On the Greater Litany' (ed. Godden, *Homilies*), ll. 246–70, and 'On the Chair of St Peter' (ed. Skeat, *Lives of Saints*), ll. 232–48; Vercelli Homily XXII; Bede, *Historia ecclesiastica*, II.1 and *Life of Cuthbert*, ch. XV; Wulfstan, Homily VI (ed. Bethurum), ll. 77–95.

[210] Ine 18, 37; Alfred 6, 25, 32; II Athelstan 14; V–VI Æthelred; II Cnut 30.1–5, 53; note also Lantfred, *Translatio et miracula*, ch. 26.

act of Christian mercy.[211] Whether any of these punishments were enacted – or, indeed, compensations extracted – is up for debate, as medieval laws are generally understood to be a record of ideals and intentions rather than strictly applied codes for judicial authorities. Regardless of enforcement, however, these texts testify to an attitude about the body and its 'missing' parts: visible impairment is associated with embarrassment, victimhood, criminality, guilt, and submission to or defeat by another.

If the impaired body in a legal context is an opportunity for the demonstration of the power of secular authority, in hagiography and didactic religious texts, it provides an opportunity for the demonstration of the power of God. As Christ heals the man blind from birth in John 9:1–7, he declares that the man is not blind because he sinned, but so that the works of God could be made manifest in him. Ælfric follows John, declaring that God has chosen the *wanhal* (*unhal*), blind, and mobility-impaired so that they can be healed and thus demonstrate his power.[212] This is the principle that undergirds the depictions of parades of impaired persons visiting holy places throughout early medieval English hagiography. A significant majority of saints' lives feature blind, deaf, non-speaking, and mobility-impaired people, as well as those mysteriously and mortally ill, cured one after the other as they handle a relic, kneel before a tomb, or pray at a shrine – a litany of fleshly miracles worked on persons portrayed as existing in a state of unremitting suffering. The impaired body reads as powerless and imperfect, and the formerly impaired body healed by contact with the saint testifies to Christian truth. Visible impairments and illnesses become a representation not only of human estrangement from heaven, but of the frailty of all flesh. All human bodies are incomplete in that no body on the postlapsarian earth can be perfect.[213] Indeed, the miraculous resurrection bodies the faithful will receive at the Last Judgement are specifically defined not only by their celestial beauty – 'ænlic ond edgeong' (peerlessly beautiful and rejuvenated), as one poem has it – but by the absence of impairment – 'hælu butan sare' (health without pain), as another poem puts it.[214] Following Augustine's declaration in his *De civitate Dei* that the sick and impaired will be made whole at the resurrection and given perfect adult bodies and minds, Ælfric insists that resurrection bodies have no *awyrdnys* (injury, damage) or *wamm* (mark, blot, stain) even for those who were *alefed* (weak) or *limleas* (limbless) in life; they will be *gehæled to ansundre* (healed to soundness).[215] Impairment itself becomes indisputable evidence of the fact that humanity is not

---

[211] O'Brien O'Keeffe, 'Body and Law', 216–17.

[212] Ælfric, 'Third Sunday after Pentecost', ll. 77–87.　　[213] Parker, 'Embodied Lives', 249.

[214] *The Phoenix* l. 53; *Christ III* ll. 1649–64. See also Vercelli Homily IV.

[215] Ælfric, 'First Sunday after Easter' (ed. Clemoes, *Homilies*), ll. 126–35.

yet reunited with God, and its healing in hagiography is a promise and a demonstration of the wholeness the faithful will experience at Judgment Day.

Yet these beatifying narratives and doctrinal sermons require impaired bodies: relics are proven true by the act of healing. An endless supply of *unhal* bodies is narratively essential, and those bodies are useful only when they are *unhal*. The numerous impaired persons in saints' lives are defined only by their impairments (the blind women, the limbless man) and appear in the narrative only to have their impairments miraculously removed from them. The pilgrim generally vanishes from the narrative immediately once healed, is left with a scar or mark indicating the 'resealing' of the body and providing a permanent reminder of the wound that was miraculously closed, or appears in a brief scene in which their kin and neighbours exclaim over their newfound ability, noting that they were once impaired and now are not. All of these narrative scenarios suspend the pilgrim in a liminal state in which their body can be neither healthy nor unhealthy, but must perpetually be both, only whole because once impaired. The Old Minster at Winchester, which contains the tomb of St Swithun, is 'eall behangen mid criccum and mid creopera sceamelum fram ende oð oþerne on ægðrum wage, þe ðær wurdon gehælede and man ne mihte swaðeah macian hi healfe up' (entirely hung with crutches and with the stools of 'cripples' who were healed there from one end to the other in either direction, and they could not put even half of them up).[216] These prosthetic devices stand in for the bodies of pilgrims, permanently preserving the sign of the *unhal* body made *hal* as a show of power legible to other visitors. The very presence of supposedly abandoned crutches at the shrine stands in for the moment of physical transformation. More broadly, the Church requires the existence of poor and impaired people in order to bestow charity, amply demonstrated in the saints' lives by stories of wealthy Christians who prove their piety by briefly adopting an impaired person and making a public spectacle of their generosity.[217] Impairment is what disability studies scholars call a *narrative prothesis*: 'a crutch upon which literary narratives lean for their representational power, disruptive potentiality, and analytical insight', seeking to expose and then rehabilitate the impaired body as a symbol of deviance.[218] In early medieval England, the impaired body signifies not deviance *per se* but original sin and the suffering of humanity, redeemed through the mercy of God, endured as a demonstration of spiritual humility, and erased at the resurrection.

---

[216] Ælfric, *Life of Swithun*, ll. 431–6.

[217] Lee, 'Abled', 42–3; for a particularly informative example, see Lantfred, *Translatio et miracula*, ch. 2.

[218] Snyder and Mitchell, *Narrative Prosthesis*, 49. For Parker's concept of 'spiritual prosthesis', see 'Embodied Lives', 107–10.

In the early medieval English literary record, the body is a text that can be read, that can be made to speak. Perceptions of impairment rest upon one base assumption that can then be interpreted in multiple ways: impairment is a lack of power and an absence of strength. That absence can provide the opportunity for healing, for a purifying ordeal, and for the intrusion of the divine, but it can also be a marker of pain, misfortune, loss, and shame. The disempowered body merits compensation and a protection that doubles as restriction in the law-codes, treatment for its recalcitrant parts in the medical texts, and access to divinity in the religious material – but only because it serves as a symbol of humanity's fallenness and estrangement from God, as a reason for pity, a cause for humility, and a source of suffering. Yet the normative body is only defined in comparison to the non-normative body. The saint's miraculous gifts are only proved by the healing of the 'cripples' and the hanging of their crutches and stools as a sign of divine transformation. The perfected resurrection body is only meaningful in contrast to the earthly body. Feverish abbesses and limping saints can only reach the profound Christian empowerment of union with God through visible, performed submission to the powerlessness of illness. The idea of health as wholeness and completion has profound theological and cultural implications revealed only through depictions and discussions of the impaired.

This Element has, thus far, drawn from a wide variety of texts to trace essential themes and cultural concepts on a grand scale. Now we must turn to the application of these concepts, and ask how an understanding of health and the body in early medieval England can help us better understand early medieval English literature and vice versa. We conclude with a case study of holy suffering and a detailed depiction of illness as martyrdom in a nexus of texts concerned with intrusion, invasion, and the protection of purified spaces: the Old English and Anglo-Latin versions of the life of St Guthlac of Crowland.

Body, Spirit, and Disease in Stories of St Guthlac: A Case Study

St Guthlac of Crowland, early medieval England's most famous hermit saint, spent years maintaining a solitary stronghold in the East Anglian fens against the incursion of ravenous demons. Eventually, however, he fell mortally ill, narrated in the poem scholars call *Guthlac B*. Guthlac endures the assault of this *untrymnes* (infirmity) with determination and joy, understanding his departure from life as a reunion with God:

> ... se dryhtnes þegn
> on elne bad, adle gebysgad,
> sarum geswenced. Ne he sorge wæg

geocorne sefan gæstgedales,
dreorigne hyge. Deað nealæcte,
stop stalgongum, strong ond hreðe
sohte sawelhus. Com se seofeða dæg
ældum ondweard, þæs þe him in gesonc,
hat, heortan neah, hildescurum
flacor flanþracu, feorhhord onleac,
searocægum gesoht.[219]

The Lord's retainer endured in fortitude, afflicted by disease,
oppressed by pains. He was not sorrowful over the
spirit-separation, sad in mind/heart, mournful in mind/heart.
Death drew near, went with stealthy (*or* thieving) steps,
strong and savage, sought the soul-house. The seventh day
came to mankind since there sank into him, hot, near the heart,
a battle-shower, a flickering force of arrows, unlocked the
life-hoard, sought it with treacherous keys.

The poet piles on metaphor after metaphor to describe what disease is doing to Guthlac's body. He is *gebysgad* and *geswenced*, two participles that mean 'afflicted, harassed, oppressed' but also refer to attacks by an enemy. The word *sar* describes pain but also mortal wounds and physical blows. Death is an unnatural sundering of the union between soul and body – the undoing and violation of two things that ought to be bound together – and an anthropomorphised warrior and a thief who seeks to break into Guthlac's flesh, to unlock his bodily container by penetrating it with a key that cracks it open. Illness is also a shower of hot arrows sinking into the saint's body, a mortal injury on an invisible battlefield. Many of these images are immediately recognisable from the medical texts discussed in previous sections. The fundamental integrity of Guthlac's flesh is at stake, the wholeness of his embodied self, and disease threatens to defeat him in ways easily interpreted as humiliating, or as forcing him into a position of submission. His controlled endurance of this painful *unhælu* and *untrymnes* – like the endurance of Alfred, Hild, or Cuthbert – purifies him, liberates him, and martyrs him all at once. Despite the proliferation of fascinating metaphors for sickness in this poem and their clear relationship to the concepts evinced by the Old English medical corpus, no published study has yet examined the portrayal of illness specifically in the Guthlac narratives. These texts – in Latin and Old English, prose and verse – collectively provide an ideal case study in early medieval English perceptions of and ideas about the body, and the differences between Latin prose and Old English poetry bring into sharp focus the vernacular vocabularies, conventions, and concepts of sickness and health that animate the literature of this period.

---

[219] *Guthlac B* ll. 1135–45.

Invasion and the Body in Guthlac Narratives

The *Anglo-Saxon Chronicle* notes the death of St Guthlac of Crowland in 714 CE; if the surviving account of his life is to be believed, he must have been born in 673 or 674. Guthlac was a Mercian aristocrat of royal blood and, in his youth, a successful warrior on the Mercian-Welsh border.[220] After experiencing a sudden revelation of his own mortality, Guthlac abandons the battlefield and the secular life and becomes a monk at the double monastery at Hrypadun (Repton). There, he learns about the eremitic saints and their solitary battles with demons in the wilderness and determines to engage in the same struggle. He builds himself a dwelling near Cruglond (Crowland) in the uncultivated, unsettled East Anglian fens, an English equivalent to the Egyptian desert that famously served as the retreat of St Paul and St Antony. Guthlac builds his new hermitage by a burial mound that has been plagued by devils, whom he banishes. He then engages in numerous battles with these demons, who assault him, attempt to reclaim the barrow, and, at one point, drag him to the mouth of Hell, where he is saved by the intercession of St Bartholomew. Guthlac becomes a respected spiritual authority and a counsellor to the future king of Mercia, Æthelbald, before he dies of an unnamed illness. A Latin prose *Life of St Guthlac* was written at the behest of the East Anglian king Ælfwald by a monk (likely also East Anglian, or living in East Anglia) named Felix, probably between 730 and 740.[221] Felix's *vita* was translated into Old English prose in the ninth or tenth century, and the portion detailing Guthlac's battles with demons is preserved separately as one of the Vercelli Homilies.[222] Two Old English poems about Guthlac also survive in the tenth-century Exeter Book miscellany: *Guthlac A* describes Guthlac's struggle with the demons, his visit to the Hellmouth, and the intercession of Bartholomew, while *Guthlac B* expands vividly on Chapter 50 of Felix's *vita* to describe Guthlac's final illness, his last preaching to his devoted servant Beccel, and his death.[223] In all its forms, the immanent Guthlac narrative revolves around the defence and regulation of both Guthlac's body and the barrow in which he dwells.

Felix drew on a number of Latin sources for his narrative, including the lives of the desert fathers and other saints known for their interactions with devils.[224] Writing (probably) in an English monastery and (undoubtedly) for an English audience, however, he arguably transformed his source material to focus on concerns about physical violation that are not present in the originals. Felix describes in great detail the devils who come to force their way into Guthlac's

---

[220] Roberts, *Poems*, 2–5.   [221] Colgrave, *Life*, 15–17.   [222] Roberts, 'Inventory', 203.

[223] On the division of the poems, see Roberts, *Poems*, 48–9; Clarke, *Writing Power*, 15–16.

[224] Thacker, 'Felix'.

hermitage and injure, damage, and break open his body. The *Life of St Antony* and other *vitae* of the eremitic saints portray demons as self-evidently psychological, representations of the saint's internal struggles. By contrast, Felix's demons are flesh and blood: they take the forms of a dozen roaring, snarling, clawing animals, assault the saint with weapons to cause physical injuries, and tow him through water and air.[225] Felix emphasises that these demonic attacks – in which Guthlac is bound, struck with iron whips, and dragged through muddy water and bramble patches – happen to the saint *corporaliter* (carnally, bodily) rather than *extra corpus*.[226] The demons also seek to re-enter and reclaim the barrow from which Guthlac has displaced them. They do not appear in the wilderness when the saint does, as in Antony's *vita*, but rather inhabit the fens prior to Guthlac's holy act of settler-colonialism. Guthlac reclaims a territory that is described repeatedly as monstrous, hellish, and estranged from God; he then reconsecrates the *tumulus* as space in which he can be in a prelapsarian relationship with nature, commanding the birds in the air and the waters of the fen to obey him.[227] The devils who previously lived there, however, constantly seek to breach these newly established bounds. The imagery is vivid:

> En subito teterrimis inmundorum spirituum catervis totam
> cellulam suam impleri conspexit. Subeuntibus enim ab
> undique illis porta patebat; nam per criptas et cratulas
> intrantibus non iuncturae valvarum, non foramina cratium
> illis ingressum negabant; sed caelo terraque erumpentes,
> spatium totius aeris fuscis nubibus tegebant. Erant enim
> aspectu truces, forma terribiles, capitibus magnis, collis
> longis, macilenta facie, lurido vultu, squalida barba,
> auribus hispidis, fronte torva, trucibus oculis, ore foetido,
> dentibus equineis, gutture flammivomo, faucibus tortis,
> labro alto, vocibus horrisonis, comis obustis, buccula
> crassa, pectore arduo, femoribus scabris, genibus nodatis,
> cruribus uncis, talo tumido, plantis aversis, ore patulo,
> clamoribus raucisonis.

> He suddenly saw the whole tiny cell filled with horrible
> troops of foul spirits; for the door was open to them as
> they approached from every quarter; as they entered
> through floor holes and crannies, neither the joints of the
> doorways nor the openings in the wattle-work denied them
> entry, but, bursting forth from the earth and sky, they
> covered the whole space beneath the heavens with their

---

[225] Felix, *Life* (ed. Colgrave), chs. 29, 31, 35, 36. All text and translations of Felix are from this edition. On Felix's demons, see Brooks, *Restoring Creation*, 200–5.

[226] Thacker, 'Felix', 11, 14–15.   [227] Brooks, *Restoring Creation*, 174–230.

dusky clouds. For they were ferocious in appearance,
terrible in shape with great heads, long necks, thin faces,
yellow complexions, filthy beards, shaggy ears, wild
foreheads, fierce eyes, foul mouths, horses' teeth, throats
vomiting flames, twisted jaws, thick lips, strident voices,
singed hair, fat cheeks, pigeon breasts, scabby thighs,
knotty knees, crooked legs, swollen ankles, splay feet,
spreading mouths, raucous cries.[228]

The depiction of devils squeezing themselves into Guthlac's cell through floor holes and door joints has no clear parallel in Felix's sources. The endless details of their physical appearances – including their human body parts, listed in a litany like those we have seen in the previous section, but made abject, animalistic, and diseased or impaired – along with the focus on the way they burst into what should be consecrated space indicates a profound anxiety around literal, physical boundary violation and penetration as a threat to both the saint's body and his Christian project. Indeed, once inside, the demons are able to seize Guthlac and subject him to the torments described earlier. Gaining access to the barrow gives them the ability to manhandle and wound his body. The saint's defence of the mound and his defence of his body are made analogous: the walls of the hermitage are equivalent to the flesh that contains Guthlac's soul. Felix continually focuses on the ways devils try to enter both human spaces and human bodies, describing instances of demon possession and influence that he explicitly likens to the ingestion of a poison that the victim must subsequently vomit up. When Guthlac experiences despair, similar to an episode in the *Life of St Antony* that describes internal struggle only, Felix turns it into a weaponised assault: Satan 'tum veluti ab extenso arcu venenifluam desperationis sagittam totis viribus iaculavit, quousque in Christi militis mentis umbone defixa pependit. Interea cum telum toxicum atri veneni sucum infunderet, tum miles Christi totis sensibus turbatus de eo' (shot, as from a bow fully drawn, a poisoned arrow of despair with all his might, so that it stuck fast in the very centre of the mind of the soldier of Christ. Now when meanwhile the poisoned weapon had poured in its potion of black venom, then every feeling of the soldier of Christ was disturbed by it).[229] Poison and supernatural arrows are, as previously discussed, favoured images in the Old English medical corpus as well as popular Hiberno-Latin *loricae*, and common in vernacular poetic depictions of the devil. Again Felix transforms his source material into a narrative that resonates with cultural concerns found specifically in the literature of the medieval North Atlantic. The Old English prose translation further describes the *geættredan stræle* (poisoned arrow) as penetrating Guthlac's *heort* (heart-organ) and *mod*.[230] *Mod* means, simultaneously, 'mind', 'spirit', and 'heart'. As discussed in what

---

[228] Felix, *Life*, ch. 31.   [229] Felix, *Life*, ch. 29.   [230] *Old English Life* (ed. Gonser), ch. 4.

follows, the vernacular early medieval English understanding of the mind locates it in the heart and treats it as a near-physical part of the chest or breast. A penetrative threat to Guthlac's mind, spirit, and self is also a threat to the body – and vice versa. Sainthood consists in the successful banishment of demons from his presence, his hermitage, and the bodies of others; sainthood is the ability to maintain inviolate boundaries.

Guthlac A's account of these demonic assaults focuses even more closely on the potential human vulnerability, and demonstrated saintly invulnerability, of Guthlac's flesh, and the fact that this concern intensifies in a vernacular, poetic text suggests the importance of the idea of the impenetrable body in the Old English literary imagination. As in Felix, Guthlac reclaims the fenland mound for God, Christianity, and humanity, and transforms this *mearclond* (lit. 'boundary-land') into paradise.[231] Just as Guthlac's *mod* is both arena and prize in a battle between an angel sent by God and a devil who seeks to prevent his Christian awakening, Guthlac 'þæt lond Gode / fægre gefreoþode' (defended that land well for God) against military troops of demons and their *færscytum* (sudden shots).[232] The demons threaten to overrun the barrow, burn him alive within his hermitage, and summon an even greater army that will trample him and carry off his wounded body, leaving only bloody tracks behind. The text continually asserts, however, that Christian power – wielded by Guthlac, by Bartholomew, and by God on Guthlac's behalf – lies in the prevention of bodily penetration. Guthlac declares, 'þeah þe ge hine sarum forsæcen, ne motan ge mine sawle gretan' (although you afflict [my body] with wounds, you cannot approach/touch/attack my soul, l. 377), and repeats constantly that the demons who assault him cannot truly injure or kill him, because his *mod* – or *hyge, breost, feorhloca*, and other words that denote the mind held within the chest – is filled up with the light and love of God. Though God permits the demons to take Guthlac in their *gifrum grapum* (greedy grips), the poem asserts that he is not hurt. When intervening for Guthlac at the entrance to Hell, Bartholomew declares:

> Ne sy him banes bryce   ne blodig wund,
> lices læla ne laþes wiht,
> þæs þe ge him to dare gedon motan,
> ac ge hine gesundne asettaþ þaer ge hine sylfne genoman.[233]

> Nor let there be breaking of bones or bloody wound, nor bruising
> of the body nor any injury, from whatever you can do to harm him,
> but you will set him down sound/whole where you seized him.

---

[231] *Guthlac A* l. 174. For a summary of previous scholarship on the barrow, see Brooks, *Restoring Creation*, 231–3.

[232] *Guthlac A* ll. 111–18, 151–2.   [233] *Guthlac A* ll. 698–702.

Bartholomew then commands the demons to 'him sara gehwylc / hondum gehælde' (heal every wound on/in him with [their] hands, ll. 704–5), suggesting that Guthlac's body has in fact been injured, despite Guthlac and the narrator's repeated insistence that he cannot be wounded. He is and is not hurt; is and is not overcome, entered, or violated. The fantasy of Guthlac's *mod* and *breost* rendered invulnerable through the presence of God's light within them – the idea that the saint has a radiant soul within his flesh-covering that cannot be touched or entered – is a fantasy of *gesundnes* (soundness), bound up with the same ideas about the body found in the medical texts and filtered through contemporary debates about the relationship between soul and flesh. Guthlac's 'blod and ban', which will be consigned to death (l. 380), are a liability; his sainthood is proven through a lack of damage, and the healing of wounds that never successfully pierced his flesh. By insisting on Guthlac's untouchability so often and in such detail, vacillating on whether or not he is physically injured, *Guthlac A* draws even greater attention to the anxiety produced by the vulnerability of normal human flesh – both despite and because of the fact that Guthlac supposedly lacks such vulnerability. The oldest English iteration of the eremitic saint is concerned in every version with boundary violation, bodily integrity, and the erasure or undoing of damage to the flesh. This is the literary context in which we read *Guthlac B*, the longest depiction of a person suffering from illness within the Old English corpus.

Guthlac's Mortal Illness

Felix's *vita* depicts a sick person in great detail – but it is not Guthlac. Offa, retainer of Æthelbald of Mercia, comes to the saint having stepped on a thorn, a wound that quickly becomes infected:

> ... inflatico tumore dimidia pars corporis ipsius a lumbis tenus plantam turgescebat. In tantum enim novi doloris molestia angebatur, ut sedere aut stare vel iacere nequisset. Nam fervente membrorum conpagine ab imis ossium medullis inmenso ardore coquebatur.

> ... half of his body was distended with a puffy swelling from the loins to the soles of the feet. And he was so sorely afflicted by the fresh pain that he was able neither to sit nor stand nor lie down. The joints of his limbs were inflamed, and he burned with an immense heat right to the very marrow of his bones.[234]

---

[234] Felix, *Life*, ch. 45.

When Offa is wrapped in Guthlac's robe, the thorn shoots out of his foot like an arrow from a bow ('velut sagitta ab arcu demissa') and his body returns to its normal proportions. The image of an arrow-like penetrative agent of pain and sickness is familiar from texts like the verse charm for a stabbing pain discussed in the second section. This affliction, too, reaches far into the body, into the bones ('ab imis ossium medullis'), even if the Latin tellingly does not refer to vernacular ideas of animate disease. Indeed, the Old English prose translation adds a highly relevant phrase, noting that when Offa is wrapped in the holy garment 'þa ne mihte þæt þæt sar aberan' (then the wound/pain could not abide it), imputing intention and agency to the sickness.[235]

Yet Felix describes almost nothing of Guthlac's illness. Using Bede's equally restrained *Life of Cuthbert* as a blueprint for the saint's death scene, all Felix tells us of Guthlac's sickness is that 'subito illum intimorum stimulatio corripuit' (a spasm of his inward parts suddenly seized him). He then repeats that the saint was seized (*arreptare*) with illness (*infirmitate*).[236] The Old English prose follows his reticence.[237] Both *Guthlac A* and the prose excerpt found in the Vercelli Book elide Guthlac's death entirely. *Guthlac A* simply declares that his soul is brought to heaven, and Vercelli Homily XXIII that he is taken up to heaven in both body and soul by St Bartholomew. This evident discomfort with Guthlac's death is of a piece with these narratives' concern with the restoration of consecrated bodies and spaces to wholeness – the penetration of the body by a malevolent force is for ordinary people like Offa to experience, not the saint. *Guthlac B*, however, devotes hundreds of lines of verse to exploring precisely this anxiety, drawing our attention – as *Guthlac A* does – to the contrast between the saint's penetrable flesh and untouchable soul.

Guthlac's disease is named as *bancoþa*, a difficult word to translate but one that only appears otherwise in the medical corpus.[238] The fact that the Old English poet uses medical language where Felix uses the more generic *infirmitate* suggests that *Guthlac B* is aware of an early medieval English vocabulary of and discourse around illness, and indeed the images the poet uses are strikingly similar to those found in medical charms. Disease is a fatal or deadly arrow (*wælstrælum, wælpilum*) or shower of arrows (*hildescurum, flacor flanþracu*) that has pierced the saint's body.[239] It is the assault of armed enemies (*feonda gewinna*) who attack (*gebysgian*) Guthlac, and death is personified as a *wiga wælgifre* (warrior greedy for slaughter).[240] The sickness is a surging heat that consumes Guthlac's body like fire, and that heat itself is presented as part of a martial struggle: 'wæs se bancofa / adle onæled ... wæs seo adl þearl, / hat ond

---

[235] *Old English Life*, ch. 16.   [236] Felix, *Life*, ch. 50.   [237] *Old English Life*, ch. 20.
[238] *Dictionary of Old English A to I* s.v. 'Bancoþa'.   [239] *Guthlac B* ll. 1143–4, 1154, 1286.
[240] *Guthlac B* ll. 961, 979, 999, 1012–13, 1136. See further Rosier, 'Death'.

heorogrim. Hreþer innan weol, born banloca' (the bone-container was ignited by disease ... the sickness was severe, hot and battle-grim. The breast boiled within, the bone-enclosure burned, ll. 954–80). Illness enters (*in gewod*) Guthlac, and indeed when death arrives, 'him duru sylfa / on þa sliðnan tid sona ontyneð, / ingong geopenað. Ne mæg ænig þam / flæsce bifongen feore wiðstondan ... ac hine ræseð on / gifrum grapum' (one soon opens the door for himself at that cruel time; the entrance opens. Nor can any enveloped in flesh resist it with life ... but it rushes on one with greedy grips, ll. 991–6). Some of these images also have liturgical parallels, but the selection and juxtaposition of these particular metaphors in a text employing medical language is especially resonant.

Sickness is also an oppressive pressure, and it fetters and binds (*gebindan*). Guthlac is *inbendum fæst* (held with inner bonds, l. 955) and his body is *legerbedde fast* (held in the sickbed, l. 1032). Multiple times, however, the poem also says that sickness or death *onleac* (unlocked) his *lichord* or *feorhhord* (body- or spirit-hoard).[241] Scholars have noted that these images seem contradictory,[242] but in the language of disease as submission, defeat, or loss of power, they need not be. Sickness seizes and binds Guthlac's body because it forces him into a position of submission; thus bound, he is also broken open and entered in an act of invasion or penetration. Other instances of the phrase *x-hord onlucan* describe a voluntary sharing of words, verse, or information; the person concerned opens their intellectual faculties to communicate with another. Here, by contrast, Guthlac's body is opened against his will. Framing illness and death in this way martyrs Guthlac – he dies in conflict with an enemy of both God and humanity, enduring that opponent's tortures until he is joyously released – but also explores the cultural anxieties surrounding sickness on a grand scale. Guthlac's bodily 'unlocking' leads to his attainment of heaven, but as with the experience of holy impairment, the assault and breaking-open is a loss of power that must be endured, to which the saint must consciously and deliberately submit. The separation of body and soul is a sundering and a curse visited upon humanity through Adam and Eve's sin (ll. 857–71), even if it does allow Guthlac's spirit to dwell with God.

The penetrability of the saint's body is counteracted by the poem's assertion – like *Guthlac A*'s – that only Guthlac's flesh-covering can be injured, and that his inner core, both his *mod* (mind/heart) and his *sawle* (soul that persists after death), are unbroken and untouched. Though sickness burns his body, Guthlac's heart also burns (vb. *beornan*) with eagerness for heaven and love for God, an answering inner heat that overcomes (vb. *forswiðan*) his pains. The poet constantly reiterates that Guthlac's untouched spirit is joyous, unafraid, and

---

[241] *Guthlac B* ll. 956, 1029, 1144.   [242] For example, Cavell, *Weaving Words*, 200–13.

unburdened by sorrow, but Guthlac also fortifies his *mod* specifically against incursion. He is 'heard ond hyge-rof' (hard and valiant of mind, l. 953) and 'he his modsefan / wið þam færhagan fæste trymede / feonda gewinna' (he securely firmed up his mind-heart against the sudden onslaught of enemies' attacks, ll. 959–61). That he makes his mind *trym* against the assault of an illness described as *untrymnes* is telling. Multiple times a description of Guthlac's physical exhaustion is paired with a description of the *heardnes* (hardness) of his *mod* or *hyge*.[243] Both *Guthlac A* and *Guthlac B* engage with this idea of a fortified, inviolate self within the body, an invulnerable core 'flæsce bifongen' (enveloped in flesh, l. 994). Guthlac's inner hardness counteracts the anxiety provoked by the assaults on the saint's physical form, an anxiety raised in Felix's Latin prose but made the nearly unremitting focus of the Old English verse. Guthlac's untouchable, contained *mod* must apparently be constantly shored up, given the poem's regular reiterations that he made his mind firm against his enemies. His sainthood consists in his perpetual refortification of his self and soul against malevolent intrusion.

Guthlac does also achieve a moment of bodily invulnerability and perfection. Death is described several times in the poem as a wrongful separation of the soul and flesh, a sundering of what should be whole,[244] but Guthlac's strength of mind promises a resurrection of the *hal* body. The poet of *Guthlac B* takes care to note that had Adam and Eve not sinned, they would not have died in Eden but rather would have been taken up to heaven 'leomu lic somud ond lifes gæst' (limbs, body, and the spirit of life together, l. 838). The poem positions Guthlac between Adam – who brought death and sickness into the world – and Christ, who 'in lichoman ... ærist gefremede' (brought about a resurrection of the body, ll. 1099–1100). The saint imitates Christ, dying at Easter after eight days, and thereby helps to redeem Adam's sin.[245] As he releases his soul to heaven, Guthlac 'his eagan ontynde, / halge heafdes gimmas ... ond þa his gæst onsende / weorcum wlitigne in wuldres dream' (opened his eyes, the head's holy gems ... and then sent his spirit, made beautiful by his deeds, into the joy of glory, ll. 1301–4). The kenning *heafod-gimm* appears elsewhere in the corpus to describe the eyes – always emphasising their value, especially in Christian bodies under threat or divine scrutiny – but juxtaposed between Adam's consignment of the body to the grave and Christ's embodied resurrection this choice of formula recalls the transfigured resurrection body, which is beautiful like 'golde and seolfre and swa þam deorwyrðestan gemcynne and eorcnanstanum' (gold and silver and like the most precious gems and pearls), according to Vercelli Homily IV.[246] At the

---

[243] *Guthlac B* ll. 545, 953, 977, 1109. See Low, 'Mental Cultivation'. [244] Rosier, 'Death', 85.
[245] Calder, 'Theme', 235; Lucas, 'Easter'.
[246] Vercelli Homily IV ll. 158–60. See *Andreas* l. 31; *Christ III* l. 1330.

exact moment of transcendence, as Guthlac's similarly transfigured and beauti-fied soul departs his body, his body is elevated into something other, and holier, than flesh. The attacking demons, by contrast, are *adloman* ('crippled' by fire).[247]

Reading *Guthlac B* in the context of the language, metaphors, and central cultural anxieties of the Old English medical texts illuminates the poem, and draws attention to the ways in which vernacular literature expands on and draws out particular anxieties around the body that the Anglo-Latin prose only begins to explore. Yet *Guthlac B* also offers us insight into another essential vernacular approach to the body, in the person of Guthlac's servant Beccel: the so-called hydraulic model of emotionality and thought.

Beccel's Emotional Body

The descriptions found throughout Old English literature of the body as a container – *bancofa, ferðloca, sawelhord* – not only interact with ideas about sickness and health but also contribute to ideas about the feeling, thinking self. These links between illness and emotion, health and self-restraint, further illumin-ate the ways the early medieval English conceived of their bodies. Pre-Conquest, vernacular descriptions of the relationship between mind, body, and soul evince a coherent and specific understanding of how the mind-in-the-body works – distinct from contemporary Platonist-Christian ideas of mind-body dualism.[248] Old English poetry and prose see the mind and heart as one corporeal entity, residing in the chest cavity. The *mod, hyge, sefa,* or *ferð* encompasses conscious-ness, rational thought, will, desire, agency, memory, and emotion. It is distinct from the *sawol,* the entirely non-corporeal part of the self that persists after death and attains heaven but participates very little in conscious life. Strong emotion or exertion of the will happens in the *mod,* and causes heat to rise around the heart and inside the chest (a concept referred to as the 'hydraulic' or 'cardiocentric' model of emotionality). Because the mind is part of the body, the heat of emotion causes physical symptoms, including swelling, chest pressure, feelings of boiling and surging within the body, and occasionally leakage like sweat, tears, or sound. The *mod* and its internal seething must be appropriately constrained by the individual: boiling emotions must often be kept inside the body-container and sealed off unexpressed. This restraint is gendered – numerous Old English texts treat it as an element of aristocratic Christian masculinity – and related to a model of the masculine body as one that penetrates and is not penetrated, a body that is

---

[247] *Guthlac B* l. 912. See also *Andreas* l. 1172, where Satan is called *hellehinca* (hell-limper).

[248] This paragraph draws on and summarises Godden, 'Mind', and Lockett, *Psychologies*, chs. 1, 2, and 4.

(ideally) closed rather than open.[249] The hydraulic model of the body thus interacts with the invasive model of illness on multiple levels. When sickness is treated as a martial defeat or sexual assault, then the experience of disease becomes – like the boiling over of emotion – a threat to the maintenance of a hegemonic masculine body. Sickness and emotion also act upon the body itself in similar ways. Illness breaks into the body from without, and (as in the case of Guthlac) can then cause surges of heat within the flesh. Emotion, too, causes heat to surge up in the body and push on its bounds from the other direction, leading to distension and leakage.

Guthlac B draws attention to precisely this correspondence. Guthlac does not experience surging or boiling within his *mod*, only a burning eagerness to enter heaven. The heat of illness seethes within his flesh, where it has inappropriately entered, but he fortifies his mind-heart against both intrusion and the inner threat that hot emotional turmoil poses to the bounds of his embodied self. Guthlac's servant, however – named as the monk Beccel in Felix, unnamed in *Guthlac B*, perhaps to render him a symbol of human grief or an allegory for the body bereft of the soul – is unable to restrain his mind-heart within his breast as his master's death approaches.[250] Beccel feels *modceare* (mind-sorrow) and is repeatedly described as grieving in his *sefa* and sad or mourning in his *hyge*. His emotion causes heat to rise in him: his sorrow is 'hatost on hreþre' (hottest in the breast, l. 1020) and he is repeatedly described as 'hat æt heortan' (hot at heart, ll. 1209, 1336). That heat also results in burning bodily leakage: 'he hate let / torn þoliende tearas geotan, / weallan wægdropan' (suffering grief, he let hot tears pour out, the drops of water surge, ll. 1055–7). Beccel's emotions are explicitly likened to the illness his master suffers, both in that he burns with emotion while Guthlac burns with disease, and in that Guthlac himself describes Beccel's boiling grief as a sickness. 'Ne beo þu on sefan to seoc' (do not be sick in heart, l. 1077), Guthlac commands his servant, and insists that 'nelle ic lætan þe / æfre unrotne æfter ealdorlege / meðne modseocne minre geweorðan, / soden sorgwælmum' (I will not let you ever become sad after my death, weary and sick in *mod*, boiled in surges of sorrow, ll. 1259–62). Guthlac's maintenance of his mind as an inviolate part of his corporeal body thus not only counteracts the penetration to which his flesh is subject but also contrasts with his servant's human weakness and the physical vulnerability caused by his lack of emotional control. Guthlac performs an idealised version of a spiritual masculinity, meeting enemies in battle and proving the impenetrability of his mind and self. Beccel is wise and able to learn from Guthlac's fortitude, but it is precisely his lack of such fortitude that draws the audience's attention to the impenetrability of the ideal, saintly body and the way

---

[249] See Karras, *Sexuality*.   [250] See Biggs, 'Unities'; Calder, 'Theme'.

in which the assault of illness provides a dramatic poetic foil to the rigorous self-control that is its opposite and spiritual antidote.

The Guthlac materials collectively illustrate the explanatory power of the medical and literary concept of the assailable container-body. Depictions of invasive illness in Felix's Anglo-Latin prose suggest the cultural currency of these ideas about sickness and the embodied self, and gesture towards their universal appeal and the points of contact they share with other intellectual traditions. The profound intensification of, and increased focus on, these themes in the vernacular texts – and in poetry specifically – shows the fascination and prominence of these ideas and anxieties about the body in the early medieval English literary and intellectual imagination. Other texts – ranging from the *Lives* of Swithun, Margaret, and Cuthbert to *Beowulf* – could benefit from such an approach. *Guthlac B*, in particular, points scholars towards productive new readings of the interactions between illness, gender, and emotion that are inherent to the understanding of the body as a sealed container, vulnerable to intrusion from without and disruption from within.

Conclusion

To ask what it means to be sick and healthy – what it means to have a body that can get sick and be restored to health – is to interrogate some of the most fundamental concepts available to a given culture in a given time period. How does a body function ideally, and how does it function in lived experience? Is the body meant to be a site of interchange with others and with the environment, or is it meant to be rigorously individuated and self-contained? What do hegemonic bodies look, act, and feel like? What are the boundaries between self and other, and how are they maintained? What is the place of humanity in the (super) natural world? How do we define and distinguish inside and outside, human and non-human, order and chaos, whole and fragment? Any literary-historical study that begins with pre-Conquest medical practice and the Old English medical corpus must grapple with themes and anxieties that undergird the entirety of the surviving Old English textual record.

The ideas of sickness, health, and bodies that we find in Old English medical texts – and which appear across the early medieval English literary corpus – are rooted in a prioritisation of the individuated and contained 'embodied self'. Power and safety are treated as equivalent to autonomy over the bounds of one's flesh and the avoidance of both intrusion and obtrusion. The actual, physical body is necessarily a site of mutual exchange with the surrounding world, and that porousness of the flesh becomes a potential source of suffering, powerlessness, and shame. Power is derived from the protection of one's mind-body complex from outside influence and penetration, the expulsion of any force that attempts to intrude, disciplined transcendence of the flesh, and the use of experiences of bodily abjection as a spiritual trial to propel the incorporeal element of the self to Christian union with God. The body is almost never treated as fundamentally dysfunctional or evil, but it is a liability, and its lack of wholeness is evidence of humanity's estrangement from the divine. The Old English corpus is marked by the fear of infection, pollution, or contamination. This literature treats both the individual human body and humanity at large as being constantly assailed by external, hostile agents – whether that agent be Grendel forcing his way into the *recedes muþan* (mouth of the hall) to rip apart and consume Danish warriors in *Beowulf*, a horde of arrow-shooting demons in the Guthlac material, or a troop of screaming women armed with invisible spears that cause internal pain. The work of preserving or reestablishing bodily health is constant, because such wholeness cannot be maintained: the body ages, sickens, receives wounds, becomes impaired, experiences violent emotion, and interacts with other bodies. Old English texts use the body to express and encode dichotomies of good and bad, powerful and powerless, healthy and sick, whole and broken open. Yet all of these literary and medicalised bodies are necessarily fragile, permeable, chaotic, and forever changing – they disrupt easy dichotomies. Is Guthlac injured by demons, or is he physically and mentally impenetrable? Are the impaired persons who make their way to St Swithun's tomb exercising their agency or seeking to remedy a fundamental lack of power? Will the sick body, in fact, 'soon be whole'? Early medieval English texts across the surviving corpus treat the body as a perpetual, ever-shifting battleground in a cosmic struggle between Christian humanity and forces inimical to God and mankind, a site of vulnerability and a vehicle for salvation.

Bibliography

Manuscripts

Cambridge, Corpus Christi College, MS 41 *(Remedies in margins)*

Cambridge, Corpus Christi College, MS 201 *(Penitential)*

London, British Library, Cotton MS Caligula A xv *(Contains two groups of remedies)*

London, British Library, Cotton MS Domitian A i *(Scientific miscellany)*

London, British Library, Cotton MS Vitellius C iii *(Herbarium Complex)*

London, British Library, Cotton MS Vitellius E xviii *(Remedies in prefatory material)*

London, British Library, Harley MS 585 *(Herbarium Complex and Lacnunga)*

London, British Library, Harley MS 1585 *(Contains illustrations of doctors)*

London, British Library, Harley MS 6258B *(Herbarium Complex)*

London, British Library, Royal MS 4 A xiv *(Contains wen charm)*

London, British Library, Royal MS 12 D xvii *(Bald's Leechbook and Leechbook III)*

London, British Library, Sloane MS 2839 *(Contains illustrations of doctors)*

London, Wellcome Historical Medical Library, MS 46 *(Single leaf of medical remedies)*

Oxford, Bodleian Library, MS Hatton 76 *(Herbarium Complex)*

Oxford, Bodleian Library, MS Junius 11 *(Contains illustrations of midwives)*

Oxford, Bodleian Library, Junius MS 121 *(Penitential)*

Oxford, Bodleian Library, MS Laud Misc. 482 *(Penitential)*

Primary

Ælfric of Eynsham. Ed. Peter Clemoes. *Ælfric's Catholic Homilies: The First Series*. Oxford: EETS/Oxford University Press, 1997.

Ælfric of Eynsham. Ed. Malcolm Godden. *Ælfric's Catholic Homilies: The Second Series*. Oxford: EETS/Oxford University Press, 1979.

Ælfric of Eynsham. Ed. John Collins Pope. *Homilies of Ælfric: A Supplementary Collection*. 2 vols. London: EETS/Oxford University Press, 1968.

Ælfric of Eynsham. Ed. and trans. Walter W. Skeat. *Ælfric's Lives of Saints*. 2 vols. London: EETS/Oxford University Press, 1966.

Ælfric Bata. Ed. Scott Gwara, trans. David Porter. *Anglo-Saxon Conversations: The Colloquies of Ælfric Bata*. Woodbridge: Boydell Press, 1997.

Asser. Trans. Simon Keynes and Michael Lapidge. *Alfred the Great: Asser's Life of King Alfred and Other Contemporary Sources*. Harmondsworth: Penguin, 1983.

Asser. Ed. William Henry Stevenson. *Asser's Life of King Alfred*. Oxford: Clarendon Press, 1904.

Bede. Eds. Bertram Colgrave and R. A. B. Mynors. *Bede's Ecclesiastical History of the English People (Historica ecclesiastica gentis Anglorum)*. Oxford: Clarendon Press, 1992.

Bede. Eds. and trans. W. Trent Foley and Arthur G. Holder. *Bede: A Biblical Miscellany*. Liverpool: Liverpool University Press, 1999.

Bede. Trans. Calvin B. Kendall. *On Genesis (In Genesim)*. Liverpool: Liverpool University Press, 2008.

Bede. Trans. Calvin B. Kendall and Faith Wallis. *On the Nature of Things and On Times (De Natura Rerum and De Temporum Ratione)*. Liverpool: Liverpool University Press, 2010.

Bischoff, Bernhard, and Michael Lapidge, eds. *Biblical Commentaries from the Canterbury School of Theodore and Hadrian*. Cambridge: Cambridge University Press, 1994.

Byrhtferth of Ramsey. Eds. Michael Lapidge and Peter S. Baker. *Byrhtferth's Enchiridion*. Oxford: EETS/Oxford University Press, 1995.

Carnicelli, Thomas A., ed. *King Alfred's Version of St Augustine's Soliloquies*. Cambridge, MA: Harvard University Press, 1969.

Chardonnens, Lászlo Sándor, ed. *Anglo-Saxon Prognostics 900–1100: Study and Texts*. Leiden: Brill, 2007.

Clayton, Mary, and Hugh Magennis, eds. *The Old English Lives of St Margaret*. Cambridge: Cambridge University Press, 1994.

Cockayne, Thomas Oswald, ed. and trans. *Leechdoms, Wortcunning, and Starcraft of Early England*. 3 vols. London: Longman, Roberts, and Green, 1864–6.

Colgrave, Bertram, ed. and trans. *Two Lives of Saint Cuthbert: A Life by an Anonymous Monk of Lindisfarne and Bede's Prose Life*. Cambridge: Cambridge University Press, 1940.

Felix. Ed. and trans. Bertram Colgrave. *Felix's Life of Saint Guthlac*. Cambridge: Cambridge University Press, 1956.

Godden, Malcolm, and Susan Irvine, eds. *The Old English Boethius: An Edition of the Old English Versions of Boethius' De Consolatione Philosophiae*. 2 vols. Oxford: Oxford University Press, 2009.

Gonser, Paul, ed. *Untersuchungen zum angelsächsischen Prosaleben des hl. Guthlac*. Heidelberg: C. Winter, 1909.

Günzel, Beate, ed. *Ælfwine's Prayerbook: London, British Library, Cotton Titus D. XXVI/ XXVII*. London: Boydell Press for the Henry Bradshaw Society, 1993.

Hanslik, Rudolphus, ed. *Benedicti Regula*. Vindobonae: Hoelder-Pichler-Tempsky, 1960.

Krapp, George Philip, and Elliot van Kirk Dobbie, eds. *Anglo-Saxon Poetic Records*. 6 vols. New York: Columbia University Press, 1931–53.

Lantfred. *Translatio et miracula Sancti Swithuni*. In *The Cult of St Swithun*, ed. Michael Lapidge. Oxford: Clarendon Press, 2003.

Liebermann, Felix, ed. *Die Gesetze der Angelsachsen*. 3 vols. Halle: Niemeyer, 1898–1916.

Morris, Richard, ed. *The Blickling Homilies of the Tenth Century from the Marquis of Lothian's Unique MS AD 971*. London: EETS/N. Trübner, 1880.

Niles, John D., and Maria A. D'Aronco, eds. and trans. *Medical Writings from Early Medieval England, Volume I: The Old English Herbal, Lacnunga, and Other Texts*. Cambridge, MA: Harvard University Press, 2023.

O'Brien O'Keeffe, Katherine. *The Anglo-Saxon Chronicle 5: MS C*. Cambridge: D. S. Brewer, 2000.

Orchard, Nicholas, ed. *The Leofric Missal*. London: Boydell Press for the Henry Bradshaw Society, 2002.

Pettit, Edward, ed. and trans. *Anglo-Saxon Remedies, Charms, and Prayers from British Library MS Harley 585: The Lacnunga*. 2 vols. Lampeter: Edwin Mellen Press, 2001.

Roberts, Jane, ed. *The Guthlac Poems of the Exeter Book*. Oxford: Oxford University Press, 2019.

Scragg, Donald G., ed. *The Vercelli Homilies and Related Texts*. Oxford: EETS/Oxford University Press, 1992.

Sweet, Henry, ed. and trans. *King Alfred's West Saxon Version of Gregory's Pastoral Care*. London: EETS/Oxford University Press, 1909.

Symons, Thomas, ed. and trans. *Regularis Concordia*. London: Nelson, 1953.

Tangl, Michael, ed. *Die Briefe des heiligen Bonifatius und Lullus*. Berlin: Weidmannsche buchhandlung, 1916.

de Vriend, Hubert Jan, ed. *The Old English Herbarium and Medicina de Quadrupedibus*. London: EETS/Oxford University Press, 1984.

William of Malmesbury. Eds. and trans. R. A. B. Mynors, R. M. Thomson, and Michael Winterbottom. *De gestis regum Anglorum I*. Oxford: Oxford University Press, 1998–9.

Williamson, Craig, ed. *The Old English Riddles of the Exeter Book*. Chapel Hill: University of North Carolina Press, 1977.

Winterbottom, Michael, and Michael Lapidge, ed. and trans. *The Early Lives of St Dunstan*. Oxford: Oxford University Press, 2022.

Wright, Cyril, ed. *Bald's Leechbook: British Museum Royal Manuscript 12D. xvii*. Copenhagen: Rosenkilde and Bagger, 1955.

Wulfstan. Ed. Dorothy Bethurum. *The Homilies of Wulfstan*. Oxford: Clarendon Press, 1957.

Secondary

Ármann Jakobsson. 'Beware of the Elf: A Note on the Evolving Meaning of *Álfar*'. *Folklore* 126 (2015): 215–23.

van Arsdall, Anne. 'Medical Training in Anglo-Saxon England: An Evaluation of the Evidence'. In *Form and Content of Instruction in Anglo-Saxon England in the Light of Contemporary Manuscript Evidence*, eds. Patrizia Lendinara, Loredana Lazzari, and Maria Amalia D'Aronco, 415–34. Turnhout: Brepols, 2007.

Arthur, Ciaran. *'Charms', Liturgies and Secret Rites in Early Medieval England*. Woodbridge: Boydell Press, 2018.

Atherton, Mark. 'The Figure of the Archer in *Beowulf* and the Anglo-Saxon Psalter'. *Neophilologus* 77 (1993): 653–7.

Ayoub, Lois. 'Old English *Wæta* and the Medical Theory of the Humours'. *Journal of English and Germanic Philology* 94 (1995): 332–46.

Banham, Debby. 'A Millennium in Medicine? New Medical Texts and Ideas in England in the Eleventh Century'. In *Anglo-Saxons: Studies Presented to Cyril Roy Hart*, eds. Simon Keynes and Alfred P. Smyth, 230–42. Dublin: Four Courts Press, 2006.

'Dun, Oxa, and Pliny the Great Physician: Attribution and Authority in Old English Medical Texts'. *Social History of Medicine* 24 (2011): 57–73.

'England Joins the Medical Mainstream: New Texts in Eleventh-Century Manuscripts'. In *Anglo-Saxon England and the Continent*, ed. Hans Sauer and Joanna Story, with Gaby Wexenberger, 341–52. Tempe: Arizona Center for Medieval and Renaissance Studies, 2011.

'Medicine at Bury in the Time of Abbot Baldwin'. In *Bury St Edmunds and the Norman Conquest*, ed. Tom Licence, 226–46. Cambridge: Cambridge University Press, 2014.

Banham, Debby, and Christine Voth. 'The Diagnosis and Treatment of Wounds in the Old English Medical Collections: Anglo-Saxon Surgery?' In *Wounds and Wound Repair in Medieval Culture*, eds. Larissa Tracy and Kelly DeVries, 153–74. Leiden: Brill, 2015.

Barley, Nigel. 'Anglo-Saxon Magico-Medicine'. *Journal of the Anthropological Society of Oxford* 3 (1972): 67–76.

Batten, Caroline R. 'Dark Riders: Disease, Sexual Violence, and Gender Performance in the Old English *Mære* and Old Norse *Mara*'. *Journal of English and Germanic Philology* 120 (2021): 352–80.

'Lazarus, Come Forth: Pregnancy and Childbirth in the Life Course of Early Medieval English Women'. In *Early Medieval English Life Courses: Cultural-Historical Perspectives*, eds. Thijs Porck and Harriet Soper, 140–58. Leiden: Brill, 2022.

Bierbaumer, Peter. *Der Botanische Wortschatz des Altenglischen*. 3 vols. Bern: H. Lang, 1975.

Biggs, Frederick M. 'Unities in the Old English *Guthlac B*'. *Journal of English and Germanic Philology* 89 (1990): 155–65.

Blair, John. *The Church in Anglo-Saxon Society*. Oxford: Oxford University Press, 2005.

Bohling, Solange. 'Death, Disability, and Diversity: An Investigation of Physical Impairment and Differential Mortuary Treatment in Anglo-Saxon England'. Unpublished doctoral dissertation: University of Bradford, 2020.

Bolotina, Julia. 'Medicine and Society in Anglo-Saxon England: The Social and Practical Context of *Bald's Leechbook* and *Lacnunga*'. Unpublished doctoral thesis: University of Cambridge, 2016.

Bonser, Wilfrid. *The Medical Background of Anglo-Saxon England: A Study in History, Psychology, and Folklore*. London: Wellcome Historical Medical Library, 1963.

Borsje, Jacqueline. 'A Spell Called *Éle*'. In *Ulidia 3*, eds. Gregory Toner and Séamus Mac Mathúna, 193–212. Berlin: Curach Bhán, 2013.

Brackmann, Rebecca. '"It Will Help Him Wonderfully": Placebo and Meaning Responses in Early Medieval English Medicine'. *Speculum* 97 (2022): 1012–39.

Brennessel, Barbara, Michael Drout, and Robyn Gravel. 'A Reassessment of the Efficacy of Anglo-Saxon Medicine'. *Anglo-Saxon England* 34 (2005): 183–95.

Brooks, Britton. *Restoring Creation: The Natural World in the Anglo-Saxon Saints' Lives of Cuthbert and Guthlac*. Cambridge: D. S. Brewer, 2019.

Brownlee, Emma. '"In the Resurrection No Weakness Will Remain": Perceptions of Disability in Christian Anglo-Saxon England'. *Archaeological Review from Cambridge* 31 (2017): 53–71.

Bruce Wallace, Karen. 'Intersections of Gender and Disability for Women in Early Medieval England: A Preliminary Investigation'. *English Studies* 101 (2020): 41–59.

Calder, Daniel. 'Theme and Strategy in *Guthlac B*'. *Papers on Language and Literature* 8 (1972): 227–43.

Cameron, Malcolm L. *Anglo-Saxon Medicine*. Cambridge: Cambridge University Press, 1993.

'Bald's Leechbook and Cultural Interactions in Anglo-Saxon England'. *Anglo-Saxon England* 19 (1990): 5–12.

'Bald's Leechbook: Its Sources and Their Use in Its Compilation'. *Anglo-Saxon England* 12 (1983): 153–82.

'The Sources of Medical Knowledge in Anglo-Saxon England'. *Anglo-Saxon England* 11 (1982): 135–55.

Cavell, Megan. *Weaving Words and Binding Bodies: The Poetics of Human Experience in Old English Literature*. Toronto: University of Toronto Press, 2016.

Clarke, Catherine. *Writing Power in Anglo-Saxon England: Texts, Hierarchies, Economies*. Cambridge: D. S. Brewer, 2012.

Crawford, Sally. 'Differentiation in the Later Anglo-Saxon Burial Ritual on the Basis of Mental or Physical Impairment: A Documentary Perspective'. In *Burial in Later Anglo-Saxon England*, eds. Jo Buckberry and Annia Cherryson, 93–102. Oxford: Oxbow Books, 2010.

D'Aronco, Maria Amalia. 'Anglo-Saxon Plant Pharmacy and the Latin Medical Tradition'. In *From Earth to Art: The Many Aspects of the Plant-World in Anglo-Saxon England*, ed. C. P. Biggam, 133–51. Amsterdam: Rodopi, 2003.

Dendle, Peter. *Demon Possession in Anglo-Saxon England*. Kalamazoo: Medieval Institute Publications, 2014.

DiNapoli, Robert. *An Index of Theme and Image to the Homilies of the Anglo-Saxon Church*. Hockwold-cum-Wilton: Anglo-Saxon Books, 1995.

Doyle, Conan. 'Anglo-Saxon Medicine and Disease: A Semantic Approach'. Unpublished doctoral thesis: University of Cambridge, 2017.

Fay, Jacqueline. 'The Farmacy: Wild and Cultivated Plants in Early Medieval England'. *ISLE* 28 (2021): 186–206.

Fowler, Roger. 'A Late Old English Handbook for the Use of a Confessor'. *Anglia* 83 (1965): 1–34.

Garner, Lori Ann. 'Deaf Studies, Oral Tradition, and Old English Texts'. *Exemplaria* 29 (2017): 21–40.

Hybrid Healing: Old English Remedies and Medical Texts. Manchester: Manchester University Press, 2022.

Gay, David E. 'On the Christianity of Incantations'. In *Charms and Charming in Europe*, ed. Jonathan Roper, 32–46. Basingstoke: Palgrave Macmillan, 2004.

Gerould, Gordon Hall. 'The Old English Poems on St Guthlac and Their Latin Source'. *Modern Language Notes* 32 (1917): 77–89.

Godden, Malcolm. 'Anglo-Saxons on the Mind'. In *Old English Literature: Critical Essays*, ed. Roy M. Liuzza, 284–314. New Haven: Yale University Press, 2002.

Grattan, J. H. G., and Charles Singer. *Anglo-Saxon Magic and Medicine: Illustrated Specifically from the Semi-Pagan Text 'Lacnunga'*. London: Geoffrey Cumberlege for the Wellcome Historical Medical Museum, 1952.

Hadley, Dawn M. 'Burying the Socially and Physically Distinctive in Later Anglo-Saxon England'. In *Burial in Later Anglo-Saxon England*, eds. Jo Buckberry and Annia Cherryson, 101–13. Oxford: Oxbow Books, 2010.

Hall, Alaric. 'Calling the Shots: The Old English Remedy *Gif hors ofscoten sie* and Anglo- Saxon "Elf-shot"'. *Neuphilologische Mitteilungen* 106 (2005): 195–209.

   Elves in Anglo-Saxon England: Matters of Belief, Health, Gender, and Identity. Woodbridge: Boydell Press, 2007.

Hall, Allan Richard. 'Investigating Anglo-Saxon Plant Life and Plant Use: The Archaeobotanical Angle'. In *From Earth to Art: The Many Aspects of the Plant-World in Anglo-Saxon England*, ed. C. P. Biggam, 101–8. Amsterdam: Rodopi, 2003.

Harrison, Freya, Aled E. L. Roberts, Rebecca Gabrilska, et al. 'A 1000-Year-Old Antimicrobial Remedy with Antistaphylococcal Activity'. *Molecular Biology & Microbiology* 6 (2015): 1–7.

Hill, Thomas D. 'Invocation of the Trinity and the Tradition of the Lorica in Old English Poetry'. *Speculum* 56 (1981): 259–67.

Hines, John. 'Practical Runic Literacy in the Late Anglo-Saxon Period: Inscriptions on Lead Sheet'. In *Anglo-Saxon Micro-Texts*, eds. Ursula Lenker and Lucia Kornexl, 29–60. Berlin: De Gruyter, 2019.

Horden, Peregrine. 'The Millennium Bug: Health and Medicine around the Year 1000'. *Social History of Medicine* 13 (2000): 201–19.

Huggins, Peter J. 'Excavation of Belgic and Romano-British Farm with Middle Saxon Cemetery and Churches at Nazeingbury, Essex, 1975-6'. *Essex Archaeology and History* 10 (1978): 29–117.

Jesch, Judith, and Christina Lee. 'Healing Runes'. In *Viking Encounters: Proceedings of the 18th Viking Congress*, eds. Anne Pedersen and Søren M. Sindbæk, 386–98. Aarhus: Aarhus University Press, 2020.

Jolly, Karen L. 'On the Margins of Orthodoxy: Devotional Formulas and Protective Prayers in Cambridge Corpus Christi College MS 41'. In *Signs on the Edge: Space, Text, and Margin in Medieval Manuscripts*, eds. Rolf H. Bremmer and Sarah Larratt Keefer, 135–84. Paris: Peeters, 2007.

Popular Religion in Late Saxon England: Elf Charms in Context. Chapel
Hill: University of North Carolina Press, 1996.

'Prayers from the Field: Practical Protection and Demonic Defence in
Anglo-Saxon England'. *Traditio* 61 (2006): 95–147.

Karras, Ruth Mazo, and Katherine E. Pierpont. *Sexuality in Medieval Europe:
Doing unto Others*. 4th ed. Abingdon: Routledge, 2023.

Kershaw, Paul. 'Illness, Power, and Prayer in Asser's Life of King Alfred'. *Early
Medieval Europe* 10 (2001): 201–24.

Kesling, Emily. *Medical Texts in Anglo-Saxon Literary Culture*. Cambridge:
D. S. Brewer, 2020.

Künzel, Stefanie. 'Concepts of Infectious, Contagious, and Epidemic Disease
in Anglo-Saxon England'. Unpublished doctoral thesis: University of
Nottingham, 2018.

Lapidge, Michael. 'The School of Theodore and Hadrian'. *Anglo-Saxon
England* 15 (1986): 45–72.

Lee, Christina. 'Abled, Disabled, Enabled: An Attempt to Define "Disability" in
Anglo-Saxon England'. *Werkstattgeschichte* 65 (2013): 41–54.

'Disability'. In *A Handbook of Anglo-Saxon Studies*, eds. Jacqueline Stodnick
and Renée Trilling, 23–38. Chichester: Wiley-Blackwell, 2012.

'Disease'. In *The Oxford Handbook of Anglo-Saxon Archaeology*, eds.
David Hinton, Sally Crawford, and Helena Hamerow, 704–26. Oxford:
Oxford University Press, 2011.

Liuzza, Roy M. 'Prayers and/or Charms Addressed to the Cross'. In *Cross and
Culture in Anglo-Saxon England: Studies in Honour of George Hardin
Brown*, eds. Karen L. Jolly, Catherine E. Karkov, and Sarah Larratt Keefer,
276–320. Morgantown: West Virginia University Press, 2007.

Lockett, Leslie. *Anglo-Saxon Psychologies in the Vernacular and Latin
Traditions*. Toronto: University of Toronto Press, 2011.

Low, Soon Ai. 'Mental Cultivation in *Guthlac B*'. *Neophilologus* 81 (1997):
625–36.

Lucas, Peter J. 'Easter, The Death of St Guthlac, and the Liturgy for Holy
Saturday in Felix's *Vita* and the Old English *Guthlac B*'. *Medium Ævum* 61
(1992): 1–16.

MacKinney, Loren. *Medical Illustrations in Medieval Manuscripts*. Berkeley:
University of California Press, 1965.

Magennis, Hugh. *Images of Community in Old English Poetry*. Cambridge:
Cambridge University Press, 1996.

Meaney, Audrey. 'Extra-Medical Elements in Anglo-Saxon Medicine'. *Social
History of Medicine* 24 (2011): 41–56.

'The Anglo-Saxon View of the Causes of Illness'. In *Health, Disease and Healing in Medieval Culture*, eds. Sheila D. Campbell, Bert S. Hall, and David N. Klausner, 12–33. Basingstoke: Macmillan, 1992.

'The Practice of Medicine in England in about the Year 1000'. *Social History of Medicine* 13 (2000): 221–37.

'Variant Versions of Old English Medical Remedies and the Compilation of *Bald's Leechbook*'. *Anglo-Saxon England* 13 (1984): 235–68.

Metzler, Irina. *Disability in Medieval Europe: Thinking about Physical Impairment during the High Middle Ages, c.1100–1400*. London: Routledge, 2006.

Fools and Idiots? Intellectual Disability in the Middle Ages. Manchester: Manchester University Press, 2016.

Mitchell, Stephen. 'Leechbooks, Manuals, and Grimoires: On the Early History of Magical Texts in Scandinavia'. *Arv: Nordic Yearbook of Folklore* 70 (2015): 57–74.

Moffett, Lisa. 'Food Plants on Archaeological Sites: The Nature of the Archaeobotanical Record'. In *The Oxford Handbook of Anglo-Saxon Archaeology*, eds. David Hinton, Sally Crawford, and Helena Hamerow, 346–60. Oxford: Oxford University Press, 2011.

Murdoch, Brian. 'Charms, Recipes, and Prayers'. In *German Literature of the Early Middle Ages*, ed. Brian Murdoch, 57–72. Rochester: Camden House, 2004.

Neville, Jennifer. *Representations of the Natural World in Old English Poetry*. Cambridge: Cambridge University Press, 1999.

O'Brien O'Keeffe, Katherine. 'Body and Law in Late Anglo-Saxon England'. *Anglo-Saxon England* 27 (1998): 209–32.

Ogura, Michiko. 'OE *Wyrm, Nædre*, and *Draca*'. *Journal of English Linguistics* 21 (1988): 99–124.

Oliver, Lisi. *The Body Legal in Barbarian Law*. Toronto: University of Toronto Press, 2011.

Olsan, Lea. 'The Inscription of Charms in Anglo-Saxon Manuscripts'. *Oral Tradition* 14 (1999): 401–19.

Orme, Nicholas, and Margaret Webster. *The English Hospital 1070–1570*. New Haven: Yale University Press, 1995.

Oswald, Dana. '*Monaðgecynd* and *flewsan*: Wanted and Unwanted Monthly Courses in Old English Medical Texts'. In *Feminist Approaches to Early Medieval English Studies*, eds. Robin Norris, Rebecca Stephenson, and Renée Trilling, 223–52. Amsterdam: Amsterdam University Press, 2022.

Parker, Leah Pope. 'Embodied Lives and Afterlives: Disability and the Eschatological Imaginary in Early Medieval England'. Unpublished doctoral dissertation: University of Wisconsin, 2019.

Paz, James. 'Magic That Works: Performing Scientia in the Old English *Metrical Charms* and Poetic *Dialogues of Solomon and Saturn*'. *Journal of Medieval and Early Modern Studies* 45 (2015): 219–43.

Porck, Thijs. *Old Age in Early Medieval England: A Cultural History.* Woodbridge: Boydell Press, 2019.

Pratt, David. 'The Illnesses of King Alfred the Great'. *Anglo-Saxon England* 30 (2001): 39–90.

Pulsiano, Phillip. 'The Prefatory Material of London, British Library, Cotton Vitellius E.xviii'. In *Anglo-Saxon Manuscripts and Their Heritage*, eds. Phillip Pulsiano and Elaine Treharne, 85–116. Aldershot: Ashgate, 1998.

Rabin, Andrew. 'Sharper Than a Serpent's Tooth: Parent-Child Litigation in Anglo-Saxon England'. In *Childhood and Adolescence in Anglo-Saxon Literary Culture*, eds. Winfried Rudolf and Susan Irvine, 270–90. Toronto: University of Toronto Press, 2018.

Richards, Mary P. 'The Body as Text in Early Anglo-Saxon Law'. In *Naked before God: Uncovering the Body in Anglo-Saxon England*, eds. Benjamin C. Withers and Jonathan Wilcox, 97–115. Morgantown: West Virginia University Press, 2003.

Roberts, Charlotte, and Margaret Cox. *Health and Disease in Britain: From Prehistory to Present Day.* Stroud: Sutton, 2003.

Roberts, Jane. 'An Inventory of Early Guthlac Materials'. *Mediaeval Studies* 32 (1970): 193–233.

Roffey, Simon. 'Medieval Leper Hospitals in England: An Archaeological Perspective'. *Medieval Archaeology* 56 (2012): 203–33.

Rosier, James L. 'Death and Transfiguration: *Guthlac B*'. In *Philological Essays: Studies in Old and Middle English Language and Literature in Honour of Herbert Dean Meritt*, ed. James L. Rosier, 82–92. The Hague: Mouton, 1970.

Rubin, Stanley. *Medieval English Medicine.* London: David & Charles, 1974.

Rudolf, Winfried. 'Anglo-Saxon Preaching on Children'. In *Childhood and Adolescence in Anglo-Saxon Literary Culture*, eds. Winfried Rudolf and Susan Irvine, 48–70. Toronto: University of Toronto Press, 2018.

Russcher, Anne, and Rolf Bremmer. 'For a Broken Limb: Fracture Treatment in Anglo-Saxon England'. *Amsterdamer Beiträge zur älteren Germanistik* 69 (2012): 145–74.

Sayer, Duncan, and Sam D. Dickinson. 'Reconsidering Obstetric Death and Female Fertility in Anglo-Saxon England'. *World Archaeology* 45 (2013): 285–97.

Shakespeare, Tom. 'The Social Model of Disability'. In *The Disability Studies Reader*, ed. Lennard J. Davis, 266–73. New York: Routledge, 2010.

Singer, Julie. 'Disability and the Social Body'. *postmedieval* 3 (2012): 135–41.

Skevington, Fay. 'The *Unhal* and the Semantics of Anglo-Saxon Disability'. In *Social Dimensions of Medieval Disease and Disability*, eds. Sally Crawford and Christina Lee, 7–14. Oxford: Archaeopress, 2014.

Snyder, Sharon L., and David T. Mitchell. *Cultural Locations of Disability*. Chicago: University of Chicago Press, 2006.

    Narrative Prosthesis: Disability and the Dependencies of Discourse. Ann Arbor: University of Michigan Press, 2000.

Storms, Godfrid. *Anglo-Saxon Magic*. The Hague: Nijhoff, 1948.

Sweany, Erin. 'Dangerous Voices, Erased Bodies: Reassessing the Old English *Wifgemædla* and Witches in *Leechbook III*'. In *Feminist Approaches to Early Medieval English Studies*, eds. Robin Norris, Rebecca Stephenson, and Renée Trilling, 253–78. Amsterdam: Amsterdam University Press, 2022.

    'The Anglo-Saxon Medical Imagination: Invasion, Conglomeration, and Autonomy'. Unpublished doctoral dissertation: Indiana University, 2017.

Talbot, C. H. *Medicine in Medieval England*. London: Oldbourne, 1967.

Thacker, Alan. 'Guthlac and His Life: Felix Shapes the Saint'. In *Guthlac: Crowland's Saint*, ed. Jane Roberts and Alan Thacker, 1–24. Donnington: Shaun Tyas, 2020.

Thompson, Victoria M. *Dying and Death in Later Anglo-Saxon England*. Woodbridge: Boydell Press, 2012.

Thun, Nils. 'The Malignant Elves: Notes on Anglo-Saxon Magic and Germanic Myth'. *Studia Neophilologica* 41 (1969): 378–96.

Treharne, Elaine M. 'A Unique Old English Formula for Excommunication from Cambridge, Corpus Christi College 303'. *Anglo-Saxon England* 24 (1995): 185–211.

Trilling, Renée R. 'Health and Healing in the Anglo-Saxon World'. *Studies in Medieval and Renaissance History* 3:13 (2018): 41–69.

Voigts, Linda E. 'Anglo-Saxon Plant Remedies and the Anglo-Saxons'. *Isis* 70 (1979): 250–68.

Voth, Christine. 'Women and "Women's Medicine" in Early Medieval England, from Text to Practice'. In *Feminist Approaches to Early Medieval English Studies*, eds. Renée Trilling, Rebecca Stephenson, and Robin Norris, 279–315. Amsterdam: Amsterdam University Press, 2023.

Wheatley, Edward. *Stumbling Blocks before the Blind: Medieval Constructions of a Disability*. Ann Arbor: University of Michigan Press, 2010.

Dictionaries and Databases

Bosworth, Joseph, and T. Northcote Toller, eds. *An Anglo-Saxon Dictionary, Based on the Manuscript Collections of the Late Joseph Bosworth and Enlarged by T. N. Toller*. Oxford: Clarendon Press, 1898–1921. https://bosworthtoller.com/.

Cameron, Angus, Ashley Crandell Amos, Antonette dePaolo Healey, et al., eds. *Dictionary of Old English: A to I Online*. Toronto: Dictionary of Old English Project, 2018. https://doe.artsci.utoronto.ca/.

Frantzen, Allen J., ed. and trans. 'Anglo-Saxon Penitentials: A Cultural Database'. www.anglo-saxon.net/penance/index.php.

Healey, Antonette diPaolo, John Price Wilkin, and Xin Xiang, eds. *Dictionary of Old English Web Corpus*. Toronto: Dictionary of Old English Project, 2009. https://doe.artsci.utoronto.ca/.

Cambridge Elements ☰

England in the Early Medieval World

Megan Cavell
University of Birmingham

Megan Cavell is Associate Professor in Medieval English Literature at the University of Birmingham. She works on a wide range of topics in medieval literary studies, from Old and early Middle English and Latin languages and literature to riddling, gender and animal studies. Her previous publications include *Weaving Words and Binding Bodies: The Poetics of Human Experience in Old English Literature* (2016), *Riddles at Work in the Early Medieval Tradition: Words, Ideas, Interactions* (co-edited with Jennifer Neville, 2020), and *The Medieval Bestiary in England: Texts and Translations of the Old and Middle English Physiologus* (2022).

Rory Naismith
University of Cambridge

Rory Naismith is Professor of Early Medieval English History in the Department of Anglo-Saxon, Norse and Celtic at the University of Cambridge, and a Fellow of Corpus Christi College, Cambridge. Also a Fellow of the Royal Historical Society, he is the author of *Early Medieval Britain 500–1000* (Cambridge University Press, 2021), *Citadel of the Saxons: The Rise of Early London* (2018), *Medieval European Coinage, with a Catalogue of the Coins in the Fitzwilliam Museum, Cambridge, 8: Britain and Ireland c. 400–1066* (Cambridge University Press, 2017) and *Money and Power in Anglo-Saxon England: The Southern English Kingdoms 757–865* (Cambridge University Press, 2012, which won the 2013 International Society of Anglo-Saxonists First Book Prize).

Winfried Rudolf
University of Göttingen

Winfried Rudolf is Chair of Medieval English Language and Literature in the University of Göttingen (Germany). Recent publications include *Childhood and Adolescence in Anglo-Saxon Literary Culture* (with Susan E. Irvine, 2018). He has published widely on homiletic literature in early England and is currently principal investigator of the ERC-Project ECHOE–Electronic Corpus of Anonymous Homilies in Old English.

Emily V. Thornbury
Yale University

Emily V. Thornbury is Associate Professor of English at Yale University. She studies the literature and art of early England, with a particular emphasis on English and Latin poetry. Her publications include *Becoming a Poet in Anglo-Saxon England* (Cambridge, 2014), and, co-edited with Rebecca Stephenson, *Latinity and Identity in Anglo-Saxon Literature* (2016). She is currently working on a monograph called *The Virtue of Ornament*, about pre-Conquest theories of aesthetic value.

About the Series

Elements in England in the Early Medieval World takes an innovative, interdisciplinary view of the culture, history, literature, archaeology and legacy of England between the fifth and eleventh centuries. Individual contributions question and situate key themes, and thereby bring new perspectives to the heritage of early medieval England. They draw on texts in Latin and Old English as well as material culture to paint a vivid picture of the period. Relevant not only to students and scholars working in medieval studies, these volumes explore the rich intellectual, methodological and comparative value that the dynamic researchers interested in England between the fifth and eleventh centuries have to offer in a modern, global context. The series is driven by a commitment to inclusive and critical scholarship, and to the view that early medieval studies have a part to play in many fields of academic research, as well as constituting a vibrant and self-contained area of research in its own right.

Elements in the Series

Printed in the United States
by Baker & Taylor Publisher Services